Manual of pulmonary function testing

GREGG RUPPEL

Assistant Director of Medical Services
St. John's Mercy Medical Center
Clinical Instructor, Maryville College
St. Louis, Missouri

SECOND EDITION
with 60 illustrations

The C. V. Mosby Company

ST. LOUIS • TORONTO • LONDON 1979

SECOND EDITION

Copyright © 1979 by The C. V. Mosby Company

All rights reserved. No part of this book may be reproduced in any manner without written permission of the publisher.

Previous edition copyrighted 1975

Printed in the United States of America

The C. V. Mosby Company
11830 Westline Industrial Drive, St. Louis, Missouri 63141

Library of Congress Cataloging in Publication Data

Ruppel, Gregg, 1948-
    Manual of pulmonary function testing.

    Includes bibliographies and index.
    1. Pulmonary function tests.   I.   Title.
RC734.P84R86   1979   616.2′4′075   78-21100
ISBN 0-8016-4209-4

C/CB/CB   9   8   7   6   5   4   3   2   1

Manual of pulmonary function testing

Preface

The primary function of the lung can be stated as twofold: first, oxygenation of mixed venous blood; second, removal of carbon dioxide from that same blood. These two functions depend on the integrity of the airways, the vascular system, and the alveolar septa. Ideally, tests designed to assess the integrity and functional relationships of these structures separately would be most appropriate. Since this is often difficult, many pulmonary function tests evaluate the status of the structural components in an indirect, overlapping way.

The evaluation of lung function is indicated for the following reasons:

1. To determine the *presence* of lung disease or abnormality of lung function
2. To determine the *extent* of abnormalities and the causative disease processes
3. To determine the *extent of disability* due to abnormal lung function
4. To determine the *progression* of the disease
5. To determine the *type* of disease or lesion
6. To determine a *course of therapy* in treatment of the particular lesion

This text will present, as concisely as possible, an explanation of the most common pulmonary function tests, the testing technique, and the significance of each test in regard to generalized disease processes. The text also lists, according to application, some of the more common testing hardware and reviews the capabilities of each type of instrument.

For this second edition, the chapter on testing regimes

now includes a section on pediatrics, which deals with the diagnosis and evaluation of disease states most common in children and adolescents (for example, asthma, cystic fibrosis, and chest deformities). This chapter also delves into bedside testing and the three main types of pulmonary function tests: ventilation, pulmonary mechanics, and matching of ventilation and blood flow. The revision also includes new material on chemical control of ventilation, airway resistance and conductance, closing volume and closing capacity, and carbon monoxide diffusing capacity. These additions are incorporated into the format of the first edition and are dicussed in terms of description, technique, and significance of each test. The discussion of carbon monoxide diffusing capacity has been expanded to include several methods for determining the $D_{L_{CO}}$. Finally, the Appendix, containing tables and formulas for prediction of normal values, has been revised and expanded to include needed sample calculations and a table of minimal spirometry standards. Selected references are offered at the end of each chapter so that unanswered questions may be easily pursued.

This manual is intended to serve as a text for students of pulmonary function testing and as a handy reference for technicians and physicians alike. The presentation of the material in this book presumes a rudimentary knowledge of pulmonary anatomy and physiology. The terminology used is that of the American College of Chest Physicians — American Thoracic Society Joint Committee on Pulmonary Nomenclature.

My special thanks to Drs. William Kistner, John Winter, and James Wiant and to Mr. John O'Brien for their encouragement and critical comments, to Miss Carol Bina for her assistance in preparation of the manuscript, and to Barbara Dokos and Ronald Gilmore for their assistance in preparation of the revised edition.

G. R.

Contents

CHAPTER ONE

Lung volume tests

VITAL CAPACITY (VC)

Description

The vital capacity is the largest volume measured on complete expiration after the deepest inspiration without forced or rapid effort (Fig. 1-1). The vital capacity is normally recorded in either liters or milliliters.

Technique

The vital capacity is measured by having the patient inspire maximally and then exhale completely into a bellows, spirometer, or similar device, with no time limit imposed on the maneuver. Vital capacity can also be measured from maximal expiration to maximal inspiration. This latter method is termed E-1, expiration to inspiration, and the former, I-E.

Significance

The normal values for vital capacities are computed as follows:

$$VC = AX - BY - Z$$

where

A = Height (cm)
B = Age (years)
X, Y, Z = Constants

Nomograms and regression equations for men, women, and children appear in the Appendix. The vital capacity may vary as much as 20% from predicted normal values in healthy individuals and may vary from time to time in the same individual, depending on the position of the body, etc. The vital

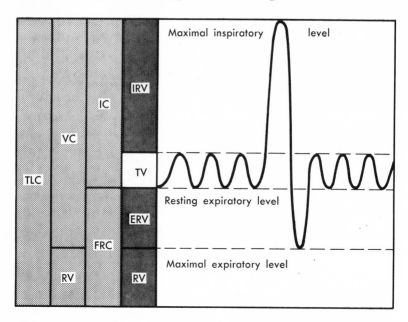

Fig. 1-1. Lung volumes and capacities. Diagrammatic representation of various lung compartments, based on a typical spirogram. *TLC*, Total lung capacity; *VC*, vital capacity; *RV*, residual volume, *FRC*, functional residual capacity; *IC*, inspiratory capacity; *TV*, tidal volume; *IRV*, inspiratory reserve volume; *ERV*, expiratory reserve volume. Shaded areas indicate relationships between the subdivisions and relative sizes as compared to the total lung capacity (TLC). The resting expiratory level should be noted, since it remains more stable than other identifiable points during repeated spirograms, hence is used as a starting point for FRC determinations, etc. (Modified from Comroe, J. H., Jr., Forster, R. E., Dubois, A. B., Briscoe, W. A., and Carlsen, E.: The lung: clinical physiology and pulmonary function tests, ed. 2, Chicago, 1962, Year Book Medical Publishers, Inc.)

capacity in adults varies directly with height and inversely with age and is generally smaller in females than in males.

A decrease in VC can be caused by a loss of distensible lung tissue, as in bronchogenic carcinoma, bronchiolar obstruction, pulmonary edema, pneumonia, atelectasis, pulmonary restriction, pulmonary congestion, or surgical excisions.

There are some causes for decreases in VC not related to lung lesions, such as depression of the respiratory centers or neuro-muscular diseases; reduction of available thoracic space by pleural effusion, pneumothorax, hiatus hernia, or cardiac en-largement; limitation of movement of the diaphragm by preg-nancy, ascites, or tumor; and limitation of thoracic movement because of scleroderma, kyphoscoliosis, or pain.

The vital capacity can be subdivided into the inspiratory capacity and the expiratory reserve volume.

INSPIRATORY CAPACITY (IC)
Description

The inspiratory capacity is the largest volume of gas that can be inspired from the resting expiratory level (Fig. 1-1). The inspiratory capacity is recorded in liters or milliliters.

Technique

The inspiratory capacity may be measured by having the patient breathe normally for several breaths and then inhale maximally while recording the changes on an appropriate spi-rogram and measuring the volume expired from the resting expiratory level. The inspiratory capacity may also be estimat-ed by subtracting the expiratory reserve volume from the vital capacity.

Significance

The inspiratory capacity normally comprises approximate-ly 75% of the vital capacity. Changes in the absolute volume of the inspiratory capacity usually parallel increases or de-creases in the vital capacity. Compensatory hyperventilation normally "dips into" the inspiratory capacity because both the end-inspiratory and end-expiratory levels are altered.

EXPIRATORY RESERVE VOLUME (ERV)
Description

The expiratory reserve volume is the largest volume of gas that can be expired from the end-expiratory level (Fig. 1-1).

Like the other lung volumes, it is recorded in liters or milliliters.

Technique

The expiratory reserve volume may be measured by having the subject breathe normally for several breaths and then exhale maximally, while recording the changes on a spirogram and measuring the volume exhaled from the average end-expiratory level. Likewise, the ERV may be estimated by subtracting the inspiratory capacity from the VC.

Significance

The expiratory reserve volume comprises approximately 25% of the vital capacity. The ERV varies greatly in comparable subjects and in the same individual with change of position. As with the inspiratory capacity, changes in the ERV are not generally of diagnostic value. Validity often depends on the ventilatory pattern of the subject.

FUNCTIONAL RESIDUAL CAPACITY (FRC) AND RESIDUAL VOLUME (RV)
Description

The functional residual capacity is the volume of gas remaining in the lungs at the end-expiratory level. The residual volume is the volume of gas remaining in the lungs at the end of a maximal expiration (Fig. 1-1). Both are recorded in liters or milliliters.

Technique

Open-circuit method. The FRC and residual volume must be measured indirectly because the RV, which is a subdivision of the FRC, cannot be removed from the lung. The concentration of nitrogen in the lungs is presumed to be in equilibrium with the atmosphere, or approximately 78%. (Actually, the N_2 concentration in the lungs is slightly less because of displacement by the respiratory gases, especially carbon dioxide and water vapor.) By having the subject breathe 100% oxygen for several minutes the nitrogen in the lungs can be gradually "washed out." The exhaled gas is collected in a spirometer or bellows and the concentration of N_2 measured; the original volume of gas in the lungs at the end-expiratory level can be computed by the following formula (see also Fig. 1-2):

$$\text{FRC} = \frac{\%N_{2_{\text{FINAL}}} \times \text{Expired volume}}{\%N_{2_{\text{ALVEOLAR}}}}$$

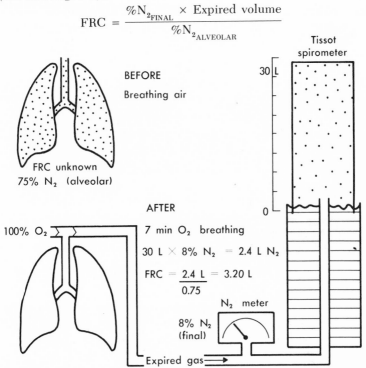

Fig. 1-2. Open-circuit determination of residual volume. In a subject breathing air the alveolar nitrogen concentration is assumed to be equal to atmospheric minus water vapor, or approximately 75%. After breathing 100% O_2 for 7 minutes and exhaling all gas into a large volume spirometer (Tissot), the entire gas sample is analyzed for N_2 concentration and the FRC computed as indicated. The switch from breathing room air to pure O_2 must come at precisely the end-expiratory level to ensure that the volume actually measured is the FRC. The residual volume is determined by subtracting the expiratory reserve volume from the FRC. (Modified from Comroe, J. H., Jr., Forster, R. E., Dubois, A. B., Briscoe, W. A., and Carlsen, E.: The lung: clinical physiology and pulmonary function tests, ed. 2, Chicago, 1962, Year Book Medical Publishers, Inc.)

where

$$\%N_{2_{FINAL}} = \text{Concentration of } N_2 \text{ in volume expired}$$
$$\%N_{2_{ALVEOLAR}} = \text{Fraction of } N_2 \text{ in alveolar gas}$$

To obtain the RV, simply subtract the ERV from the FRC as just measured. Corrections for the amount of N_2 washed out of the blood and tissue and for small amounts of nitrogen in "pure" O_2 must be made when computing the FRC. For each minute of oxygen breathing, approximately 40 ml of N_2 are removed from blood and tissue, so that a factor of 0.04 *(T)*, where *T* is time of the test, is subtracted from the derived value. The FRC must be corrected to BTPS. (See the Appendix.)

A newer method for performing the open-circuit procedure uses a rapid N_2 analyzer coupled to a spirometer or pneumotach to provide a "breath-by-breath" analysis of N_2 washed out of the lungs. Electronic signals proportional to N_2 concentration and volume (or flow) are integrated to derive the exhaled volume of N_2 for each breath, and then the values for all breaths are summed to provide a total volume of N_2 washed out. The test is continued for 7 minutes or until the $\%N_2$ in alveolar gas has been reduced to less than 1%. FRC is calculated as for the conventional method by dividing the N_2 volume by the fractional concentration of alveolar N_2 at the beginning of the test and making the necessary corrections (blood/tissue washout, temperature). In addition, a breath-by-breath plot of the $\%N_2$ (or log $\%N_2$) versus volume or number of breaths can be obtained to derive indices of the distribution of ventilation. (See Fig. 4-2.)

Closed-circuit method. The FRC can also be calculated indirectly by diluting the gas in the lungs with a gas of known concentration. A suitable spirometer is filled with a known volume of gas to which helium (or oxygen or hydrogen) has been added. The amount and concentration of helium is measured, usually about 10%, and recorded before the test is begun. Then the subject rebreathes the gas in the spirometer, with a CO_2 absorber in place, until the concentration of helium falls to a stable level, usually less than 7 minutes. If a small amount of helium is diluted in a small quantity of gas, usually 1 to 2 liters, equilibration of the helium in the lungs' rebreathing system takes place rather quickly. The final concentration of helium is then recorded. The volume that was in the spirometer before the test was begun can then be calculated:

$$\text{Initial volume} = \frac{\text{He added (ml)}}{\% \text{He}_{\text{initial}}}$$

Once the initial volume is known, the FRC (and RV) can be computed:

$$\text{FRC} = \frac{(\% \text{HE}_{\text{initial}} - \% \text{HE}_{\text{final}})}{\% \text{HE}_{\text{final}}} \times \text{Initial volume}$$

again

$$\text{RV} = \text{FRC} - \text{ERV}$$

To correct for the volume of He absorbed by the blood during rebreathing, a volume of 100 ml is usually subtracted from the FRC. The FRC must be converted to BTPS (Fig. 1-3). Sample equations for both the open- and closed-circuit techniques can be found in the Appendix.

Significance

In both the open- and closed-circuit techniques, the residual volume is measured indirectly as a subdivision of the functional residual capacity. This is the preferred method because the end-expiratory level is more constant than the points of complete inspiration or complete expiration. The end-expiratory level varies more in subjects with emphysema and thus may affect the calculation of the FRC. The validity of both the open- and closed-circuit techniques depends on the assumption that all parts of the lung are reasonably well ventilated. In patients with obstructive disease the 7-minute test period may not be long enough to wash N_2 out or mix He to a stable level in the poorly ventilated parts of the lung. Hence the FRC, RV, and all calculated volumes (TLC, ERV) will appear less than the true values. Prolongation of the test improves results

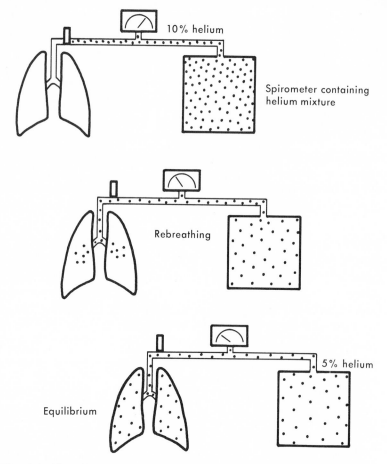

Fig. 1-3. Closed-circuit determination of residual volume. The lungs of a subject breathing air contain no helium. The subject then rebreathes a mixture of He and air or O_2, whose volume and He% are known. Helium is diluted until an equilibrium is reached. The volume of He initially present is known from the initial concentration and the volume of the rebreathing system. At the end of the test the same volume of He is now diluted in a larger volume (rebreathing system + lungs), and the total volume is computed from the initial He volume and the final He concentration:

$$\frac{V_{He_{initial}}}{\%_{He_{final}}} = \text{Total volume of system}$$

The FRC is derived by subtracting the rebreathing system volume (see text). The switch from air to the He mixture must be made at the end-expiratory level for accurate measurement of FRC. RV is derived by subtracting the ERV. (Modified from Comroe, J. H., Jr., Forster, R. E., Dubois, A. B., Briscoe, W. A., and Carlsen, E.: The lung: clinical physiology and pulmonary function tests, ed. 2, Chicago, 1962, Year Book Medical Publishers, Inc.)

somewhat but will not account for "completely" trapped gas, as found in bullous emphysema.

An increase in the FRC is normally considered pathologic. An increased FRC represents *hyperinflation*, which may result from emphysematous changes, asthmatic or fibrotic bronchiolar obstruction, compensation for surgical removal of lung tissue, or thoracic deformity. An increase in FRC results in muscular and mechanical inefficiency.

An increase in RV indicates that in spite of maximal expiratory effort, the lungs still contain an abnormally large amount of gas. This type of change appears in young asthmatics and is usually reversible. Increases of RV are also characteristic of emphysema and chronic air trapping, as well as chronic bronchial obstruction. RV and FRC usually increase together, although this is not always true. The RV may increase without loss of ability to ventilate adequately.

FRC and RV may also be decreased in diseases that occlude many alveoli, such as pneumonia.

FRC and RV are typically decreased in restrictive diseases, particularly those associated with extensive fibrosis such as sarcoidosis, asbestosis, and silicosis.

Table 1 lists typical values for lung volumes for a normal adult male, a patient with hyperinflation (as might be seen in emphysema), and a patient with restriction (as might be seen in sarcoidosis).

Table 1. Typical lung volumes for normal adult male, patient with hyperinflation and patient with restriction

Value	Normal	Hyperinflation	Restriction
VC (ml)	4800	3000	3000
FRC (ml)	2400	3600	1500
RV (ml)	1200	3000	750
TLC (ml)	6000	6000	3750
RV/TLC %	20%	50%	20%

THORACIC GAS VOLUME (V_{TG})
Description

The thoracic gas volume measures the volume of gas contained in the thorax, whether in communication with open airways or trapped in any compartment of the thorax. The thoracic gas volume is recorded in liters or milliliters.

Technique

The thoracic gas volume is measured using the body plethysmograph (Fig. 1-4). The technique is based on Boyle's

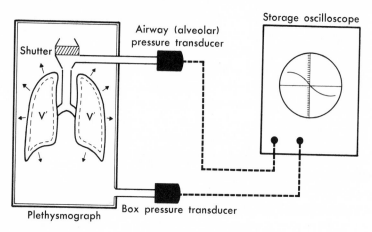

Fig. 1-4. Thoracic gas volume (V_{TG}). The body plethysmograph is used to measure thoracic gas volume. Boyle's law states that the volume varies inversely with the pressure if the temperature is held constant. The plethysmograph, with pressure transducers for measurements of box pressure and airway (alveolar) pressure, is illustrated. An electronic shutter momentarily occludes the airway so that airway pressure is approximately equal to alveolar pressure. Simultaneously, the alveolar gas is decompressed because of enlargement of the thorax, without gas flow. This change in alveolar volume and pressure is reflected by an increase in box pressure, and an estimation of the volume change can be derived by calibration. When the original pressure (P), the new pressure (P′), and the new volume (V′ or V + ΔV) are known, the original volume (V or TGV) can be computed from Boyle's law. (See text and Appendix.)

law that the volume of gas varies inversely in proportion to the pressure to which it is subjected. At the start of the test, the subject has an unknown volume of gas in the thorax. By occluding the airway and allowing the subject to decompress the gas in the chest by making an inspiratory effort, a new volume and a new pressure are generated. The change in pulmonary gas pressure is easily measured at the airway since mouth pressure equals alveolar pressure when there is no airflow. The change in pulmonary gas volume is measured by monitoring the pressure in the plethysmograph. The manometer recording box pressure is calibrated directly in terms of volume change by introducing a small, known volume of gas into the plethysmograph with the subject in place and noting the pressure change.

As the subject breathes against the closed airway, which has been occluded by means of an electrical shutter, he alternately compresses and decompresses the air within his chest by the action of his ventilatory muscles. The manometer recording mouth pressure (which equals alveolar pressure) is plotted on the vertical axis of an oscilloscope, while the manometer recording box pressure (which is calibrated as volume change) is plotted on the horizontal axis (Fig. 1-4). Changes in each parameter are graphed continuously and appear as a sloping line, which is equal to $\Delta P/\Delta V$, where ΔP equals change in alveolar pressure and ΔV equals change in alveolar volume. (The change in alveolar volume is measured indirectly by noting the reciprocal change in plethysmograph volume.)

The original thoracic gas volume can then be obtained from the slope of the tracing by applying a derivation of Boyle's law:

$$V_{TG} = \frac{P_B}{\lambda V_{TG}}$$

where

V_{TG} = Thoracic gas volume
P_B = Barometric pressure minus water vapor pressure
λV_{TG} = Slope of the oscilloscope trace equal to $\Delta P/\Delta V$

For the complete derivation of the equation, see the Appendix.

The measurements are usually made with the subject panting, with an open glottis. This type of breathing allows smaller pressure changes to be recorded at or near FRC. If the mouth shutter is closed at precisely end-expiration, V_{TG} equals FRC. Several determinations can be made quickly to obtain an average for the slope of $\Delta P/\Delta V$.

Significance

The thoracic gas volume is a quick and precise means of measuring FRC and total lung capacity. Its obvious advantage is that it measures the volume of gas in the thoracic cavity whether it is in ventilatory communication with the atmosphere or not. Hence the thoracic gas volume measurement of FRC is often larger than the FRC as measured by helium dilution or nitrogen washout, especially in severe emphysema or in closed pneumothorax. When dilution tests are extended beyond 7 minutes, the results for FRC determinations approach the thoracic gas volums figure. Normal lungs, however, show similar results by either method.

The main disadvantage of thoracic gas volume determinations is the necessity of a body plethysmograph and the requisite instrumentation.

TOTAL LUNG CAPACITY (TLC)
Description

The total lung capacity is the amount of gas contained in the lungs at the end of a maximal inspiration. It is measured in liters or milliliters.

Technique

The total lung capacity is normally calculated by combination of other specific lung volumes. The two most common are addition of the FRC and inspiratory capacity and addition of the vital capacity and the residual volume.

Determination of TLC can be performed using standard

posterior-anterior and lateral x-ray films of the chest made at a distance of 72 inches and subdividing the films into segments. The dimensions of each segment are measured and the values used to determine the segmental volumes, which are then summed. From this total thoracic volume, the volumes for the heart and diaphragms are subtracted, as well as corrections for blood and tissue volumes of the lungs themselves. This technique correlates well with plethysmographic determintions of TLC and is more accurate than gas dilution methods in cases of moderate to severe obstruction.

Significance

The TLC is decreased in edema, atelectasis, neoplasms, or restrictive lesions and in pulmonary congestion, pneumothorax, or thoracic restriction. TLC may be normal or increased in bronchiolar obstruction with hyperinflation and in emphysema. (See Table 1.) Normal or increased total lung capacity does not mean that ventilation or surface area for diffusion is normal. (For predicted normals, see the Appendix.)

RESIDUAL VOLUME/TOTAL LUNG CAPACITY RATIO (RV/TLC × 100)

Description

The RV/TLC ratio is a statement of the fraction of the total lung capacity that can be defined as residual volume, expressed as a percentage.

Technique

Divide the residual volume by the total lung capacity and multiply by 100.

Significance

In healthy young adults the RV/TLC may vary from 20% to 35%. Since this is a ratio, values greater than 35% may derive from absolute increases of the RV, as in emphysema, or from a decrease in the total lung capacity, as in restrictive diseases. Values greater than 35% do not indicate disability but are of greatest diagnostic value when correlated to the absolute values of RV and TLC. A large RV/TLC in the presence of an increased TLC is often indicative of chronic air trapping. (See Table 1).

SELECTED BIBLIOGRAPHY

Altman, P. L., and Dittmer, D. S., editors: Respiration and circulation, Bethesda, Md., 1971, Federation of American Societies for Experimental Biology.

Briscoe, W. A.: Lung volumes. In Fenn, W. O., and Rahn, H., editors: Handbook of physiology — respiration II, Washington, D.C., 1965, American Physiological Society.

Comroe, J. H., Jr., Forster, R. E., Dubois, A. B., Briscoe, W. A., and Carlsen, E.: The lung: clinical physiology and pulmonary function tests, ed. 2, Chicago, 1962, Year Book Medical Publishers, Inc.

Dubois, A. B., Bothelo, S. Y., Bedell, G. H., Marshal, R., and Comroe, J. H.: A rapid plethysmographic method for measuring thoracic gas volume: a comparison with a nitrogen washout method for measuring functional residual capacity in normal subjects, J. Clin. Invest. **35:**322, 1956.

Hickam, J. B., Blair, E., and Frayser, R.: An open circuit helium method for measuring functional residual capacity and defective intrapulmonary gas mixing, J. Clin. Invest. **33:**1277, 1954.

Kory, R. C., Callahan, R., Boren, H. G., and Syner, J. C.: The Veterans Administration – Army Cooperative Study of Pulmonary Function. I. Clinical spirometry in normal men, Am. J. Med. **30:**243, 1961.

Needham, C. D., Rogar, M. D., and McDonald, J.: Normal standards for lung volumes, intrapulmonary gas mixing, and maximum breathing capacity, Thorax **9:**313, 1954.

West, J. B.: Pulmonary pathophysiology: the essentials, Baltimore, 1977, The Williams & Wilkins Co.

West, J. B.: Respiratory physiology: the essentials, Baltimore, 1974, The Williams & Wilkins Co.

Whitfield, A. G., Waterhouse, J. A. H., and Arnott, W. M.: Subdivisions of lung volume: normal standards, Br. J. Soc. Med. **4:**1, 1950.

CHAPTER TWO

Ventilation tests

TIDAL VOLUME (V_T)

Description

The tidal volume is the volume of gas inspired or expired during each respiratory cycle, usually measured in milliliters (Fig. 1-1).

Technique

The tidal volume can be measured directly by simple spirometry. The subject breathes into a bellows or spirometer, and the volume change is measured from the excursions directly or recorded on an appropriate spirogram. Since no two breaths are identical, the tidal volume inhaled or exhaled should be measured for at least 1 minute and then divided by the rate to determine the average tidal volume:

$$V_T = \dot{V}/f$$

where

$\dot{V}$ = Volume expired or inspired over given interval
f = Number of breaths for same interval

Significance

Average values for healthy adults fall between 400 and 700 ml, but there is considerable variation even from these values. Decreased tidal volumes occur in many types of pulmonary disorders, although many patients with pulmonary disease exhibit increased tidal volumes. Tidal volume itself is not an adequate indicator of alveolar ventilation and should never be considered outside the context of rate and minute volume.

Rapid rates and small tidal volumes are often indicative of hypoventilation but must be correlated with arterial blood gas values to be definitive.

RATE (f)
Description

The respiratory rate is the number of breaths per unit of time, usually per minute.

Technique

The rate may be determined by counting the chest movements or the excursions of a bellows or spirometer for an appropriate interval. Counting the rate for several minutes and taking an average per minute is preferred to counting the rate for 10 or 20 seconds and extrapolating.

Significance

Increased or decreased rate is commonly assumed to be a sign of the ventilatory status, although its value as an index of ventilation lies solely in conjunction with measurements of tidal volume, minute volume, and arterial blood gas values. Hypoxia and hypercarbia, as well as acidosis, cause increases in respiratory rate, but an increased rate itself is not definitive. Decreased rate is common in central nervous system depression and in CO_2 narcosis.

MINUTE VOLUME ($\dot{V}_E$)
Description

The minute volume is the total volume of gas either inspired or expired in 1 minute. It includes both the alveolar and dead space ventilation and is recorded in liters per minute.

Technique

The minute volume may be determined by allowing the subject to breathe either into or out of a bellows, spirometer, or similar metering device for at least 1 minute. Measuring expired or inspired gas volume for a period of several minutes and dividing by the time gives an average minute volume. The expired minute volume is usually slightly smaller than the inspiratory because of the respiratory exchange ratio. Normally this difference is negligible. BTPS corrections should be made.

Significance

The minute volume is the best index of ventilation when used in conjunction with blood gas values. Since the $\dot{V}_E$ is the sum of both the dead space and effective alveolar ventilation, absolute values for minute volume are not necessarily indicative of hypoventilation or hyperventilation. A large minute volume may be the result of an enlarged dead space volume. Normal minute ventilation ranges from 5 to 10 L/min, with wide variations in normal subjects. Minute volume increases in response to hypoxia, hypercarbia, and acidosis and decreases in the opposite conditions. Subjects with increased respiratory dead space may exhibit minute volumes in excess of 20 L/min because a large total ventilation is necessary to ensure an adequate alveolar ventilation.

CHEMICAL CONTROL OF VENTILATION
Description

CO_2 response is the measurement of the increase or decrease in minute ventilation ($\dot{V}_E$) caused by breathing various concentrations of CO_2 under normoxic conditions ($P_{a_{O_2}} = 100$ mm Hg). It is recorded as ΔL/min/mm Hg P_{CO_2}.

O_2 response is the measurement of the increase or decrease in minute ventilation ($\dot{V}_E$) caused by breathing various concentrations of O_2 under isocapneic conditions ($P_{a_{CO_2}} = 40$ mm Hg).

Occlusion pressure (P_{100}) is the pressure generated in the proximal airway during the first 100 msec of breathing against an occluded airway, measured in cm H_2O.

Technique

CO_2 response can be measured in two ways:
1. The open-circuit technique, in which various con-

centrations (1% to 7%) of CO_2 in air or oxygen are breathed until a steady state is reached. Measurements of end-tidal P_{CO_2}, arterial P_{CO_2}, P_{100}, and $\dot{V}_E$ are then made at each concentration.

2. The closed-circuit technique, in which the subject rebreathes from a one-way circuit containing a reservoir for 7% CO_2 in O_2 (Fig 2-1), valves and pressure taps for monitoring P_{100}, and ports for extracting gas samples for end-tidal P_{CO_2} determinations. A pneumotach (see Chapter 8) is placed in line to record $\dot{V}_E$. Changes in $\dot{V}_E$ and P_{ACO_2} (end-tidal) are monitored and plotted to obtain a response curve.

O_2 response can be measured by either open- or closed-circuit techniques:

1. Open-circuit technique. The subject breathes gas mixtures containing oxygen concentrations from 12% to 20%, to which CO_2 is added to maintain the alveolar P_{CO_2} at a constant level. Once a steady state is reached, arterial P_{O_2}, $\dot{V}_E$, and P_{100} can be measured. This procedure is repeated at various O_2 concentrations to produce the response curve. (This procedure is often called a *step test*.) Continuous monitoring of end-tidal CO_2 is necessary to titrate the addition of CO_2 to the system to maintain isocapnia. Arterial P_{O_2} must be monitored since it often varies from the alveolar P_{O_2}. CO_2 response curves are sometimes measured at widely varying P_{aO_2}s, and the subsequent difference in ventilation or P_{100} at any particular P_{CO_2} is attributed to the response to hypoxemia.

2. Closed-circuit technique (progressive hypoxemia). The subject rebreathes from a system similar to that used for closed-circuit CO_2 response, but which contains a CO_2 remover. CO_2 can be added to the inspired gas to maintain isocapnia. Response to decreasing inspired P_{O_2} is monitored by recording $\dot{V}_E$ or P_{100}, and the arterial P_{O_2} or saturation is measured either directly by indwelling catheter or by ear oximetry.

P_{100} is measured using a system similar to that in Fig. 2-1. A pressure tap at the proximal airway records pressure changes versus time on a storage oscilloscope. A large bore stopcock or electronic shutter mechanism is included in the

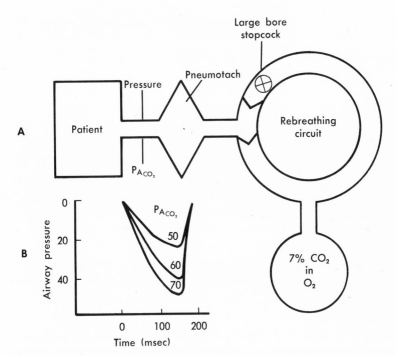

Fig. 2-1. A, Apparatus for measurement of occlusion pressure (P_{100}). A rebreathing circuit is diagrammed, which can be used for measurement of occlusion pressure and ventilation during progressive hypercapnia. Hypercapnia is produced at full arterial saturation by rebreathing 7% CO_2 in O_2 from a reservoir. Ventilation is measured by integration of the signal from the pneumotach. P_{ACO_2} and pressure are monitored from taps at the patient mouthpiece. A large-bore stopcock is placed in the inspiratory line to occlude flow for single breaths. One-way valves allow the large-bore stopcock to be closed during expiration so that the subsequent inspiration occurs against the occluded airway at FRC. **B,** Representative tracings of the airway pressure developed during occlusion at various levels of hypercapnia (P_{ACO_2} 50, 60, 70) for the first 100 msec.

inspiratory line so that inspiratory flow can be randomly occluded. The unidirectional breathing circuit allows the stopcock or shutter to be closed during expiration, so that the subsequent inspiration can occur against complete occlusion starting at FRC.

Significance

The response to an increase in P_{CO_2} in the normal individual is a linear increase in minute ventilation on the order of 3 L/min/mm Hg (P_{CO_2}). It should be noted, however, that wide variations (1 to 6 L/min) exist in normal subjects and some variation is present in repeated testing of the same individual. The response to CO_2 in patients with obstructive disease may be reduced; this is partially attributable to increased airway resistance, which has been shown to reduce ventilatory response in normal individuals. It is not yet clear why some patients with obstructive disease increase ventilation to maintain a normal P_{CO_2}, while others tolerate an increased P_{CO_2}.

The response to a decrease in $P_{a_{O_2}}$ in the normal individual appears to be exponential once the $P_{a_{O_2}}$ has fallen to the range of 40 to 60 mm Hg. Again there are wide variations in responses among individuals. The hypoxic response is increased in the presence of hypercarbia and decreased in hypocarbia. Patients with chronic obstructive lung disease and chronic CO_2 retention receive their primary respiratory stimulus via the hypoxemic response and may suffer severe or even fatal respiratory depression if that response if obliterated by uncontrolled oxygen therapy.

Some subjects with little intrinsic lung disease show markedly decreased response to hypoxemia or hypercarbia. These include patients with myxedema, obesity-hypoventilation syndrome, and idiopathic hypoventilation. CO_2 and O_2 response measurements, along with tests of pulmonary mechanics, may be particularly valuable in the evaluation and treatment of these types of patients.

Occlusion pressure has been suggested as a measurement of ventilatory response independent of the mechanical properties of the lung. Since no airflow occurs during occlusion of the airway, significant interference from mechanical abnormalities, such as increased resistance or decreased compliance, is omitted. Reflexes from the airways and chest wall are also of little influence during the first 100 msec. Therefore, the pressure generated can be viewed as proportional to the neural output of the medullary centers. This proportionality may be influenced by other factors, however, such as body position and the contractile properties of the respiratory muscles.

Occlusion pressure has been shown to increase in hypercapnia and hypoxia and appears to correlate well with the observed ventilatory responses. Some patients with chronic airway obstruction demonstrate little or no increase in P_{100} in response to an increase in their P_{CO_2}, even with increased airway resistance, whereas normal subjects do increase their P_{100} when breathing through artificial resistance, on challenge with high P_{CO_2} or low P_{O_2}. This failure to respond to increased resistance in the airways may predispose patients with chronic obstructive pulmonary disease (COPD) to respiratory failure when lung infections occur. Measurement of occlusion pressure may prove valuable in planning treatment of patients with abnormal ventilatory responses.

RESPIRATORY DEAD SPACE (V_D)
Description

Respiratory dead space is that volume of the lungs that is ventilated but not perfused by pulmonary capillary blood flow. The dead space can be subdivided into the conducting airways, or anatomic dead space, and the nonfunctioning alveoli, or alveolar dead space. The combination of alveolar and anatomic dead space volumes is the physiologic, or respiratory, dead space. Respiratory dead space is recorded in milliliters.

Technique

The respiratory dead space can be calculated in two ways. The first uses Bohr's equation defining respiratory dead space.

$$V_D = \frac{(F_{A_{CO_2}} - F_{E_{CO_2}})}{F_{A_{CO_2}}} V_E$$

where

V_E = Expired volume (tidal volume)
$F_{A_{CO_2}}$ = Fraction of CO_2 in alveolar gas
$F_{E_{CO_2}}$ = Fraction of CO_2 in expired gas

Since the concentration of CO_2 in the alveoli is difficult to measure, the partial pressures of the component gases may be substituted and the equation written thus:

$$V_D = \frac{(P_{a_{CO_2}} - P_{E_{CO_2}})}{P_{a_{CO_2}}} V_E$$

where

$P_{a_{CO_2}}$ = Arterial P_{CO_2}
$P_{E_{CO_2}}$ = P_{CO_2} of expired gas sample

Note that the arterial P_{co_2} is used in place of the alveolar P_{CO_2}, presuming of course that equilibration is perfect between the alveoli and pulmonary capillaries. The test derives from the fact that there is practically no CO_2 in the atmosphere, and therefore the partial pressure of CO_2 in the expired gas is inversely proportional to the physiologic or respiratory dead space. By collecting gas over several respiratory cycles and obtaining simultaneous arterial P_{co_2}, all the variables are supplied and a reasonably accurate physiologic dead space calculation can be made by application of the equation just given. The estimation becomes more accurate as more expired gas is collected. The accuracy depends on the measurement of V_E, as well as the partial pressure of CO_2.

A second method available for calculating the anatomic dead space is called the *single-breath analysis method*. This technique requires continuous analysis of the concentration of nitrogen in the expired gas plus simultaneous measurement of the expired volume. After inhalation of 100% O_2, the subject breathes out through the recording apparatus. During the first part of the breath pure O_2 is exhaled, and the N_2 concentration remains zero (Fig. 2-2) until a volume equal to the anatomic dead space has been exhaled. Then the N_2 concentration rises rapidly to the level of alveolar N_2, diluted with O_2. Since alveolar gas mixes with dead space gas during exhalation, the curve depicting the change in N_2 concentration does not present a "square front." By numerical methods a square front can be constructed, and the anatomic dead space is the volume expired up to the square front. Bohr's equation can be modified to apply to the data obtained from a single-breath analysis:

$$V_D = \frac{(F_{A_{N_2}} - F_{E_{N_2}})}{F_{A_{N_2}}} V_E$$

where

V_E = Expired volume

$F_{A_{N_2}}$ = Fraction of N_2 in alveolar gas (read from N_2 meter at end of breath)

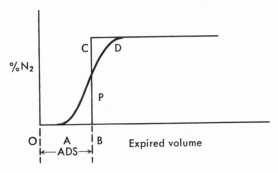

Fig. 2-2. Anatomic dead space determination. The rise in concentration of nitrogen during a single expiration, after a breath of 100% O_2, is illustrated. Only the initial portion of the breath is included. As the subject expires, the N_2 concentration rises slowly at first as pure dead space gas is exhaled; then as mixed bronchial and alveolar air is expired, the N_2 concentration rises abruptly. Since different parts of the lung empty at different rates, the change from pure dead space air to alveolar gas appears as an S-shaped curve. By constructing a square wave front *(BC)* so that the areas *ABP* and *DCP* are equal, the anatomic dead space can be estimated as equal to the volume expired up to point *B*.

$F_{E_{N_2}}$ = Fraction of N_2 in expired sample (computed by measuring area under $\%N_2$ curve and dividing by V_E)

The difficulty in obtaining the $F_{E_{N_2}}$ restricts this type of calculation to more sophisticated laboratory setups.

Significance

The measurement of respiratory dead space, although difficult, yields important information regarding the status of the functional lung capacity. The anatomic dead space is larger in men than in women as well as with increases in tidal volume caused by exercise or pulmonary disease. The anatomic dead space increases in patients with large FRCs and in diseases such as bronchiectasis. It may be decreased in asthma or in diseases characterized by bronchial obstruction. Because of the difficulty in measuring the anatomic dead space, estimates based on age, sex, and FRC may be used; for clinical purposes the anatomic dead space is sometimes equated with the subject's weight in pounds.

More important is the measurement of physiologic dead space, which is accomplished reasonably well by appliction of the Bohr equation. The volume of ventilation, which is wasted on the conducting airways and nonfunctioning alveoli, is usually expressed as a fraction of the tidal volume, V_D/V_T, and is considered normal if the derived value is 0.2 to 0.4 Expressing dead space in this way eliminates the necessity of measuring the volume of expired gas in the application of the Bohr equation. Physiologic dead space measurements are a good index of ventilation/blood flow ratios, since all CO_2 in expired gas comes from perfused alveoli. (See Chapter 6.)

ALVEOLAR VENTILATION ($\dot{V}_A$)
Description

The alveolar ventilation is that volume of gas that participates in gas exchange in the lungs and can be considered equal to the tidal volume minus the respiratory dead space. The alveolar ventilation is usually expressed as volume per unit time, normally liters per minute.

Technique

The alveolar ventilation per minute can be calculated in two ways:

1.
$$\dot{V}_A = f(V_T - V_D)$$

where

V_T = Tidal volume
V_D = Respiratory dead space
f = Respiratory rate

Often, for the sake of convenience, the respiratory dead space is estimated as equal to the anatomic dead space. This method is valid only when the inspired gas is uniformly distributed in relation to pulmonary blood flow.

2. Since atmospheric gas contains almost no CO_2 alveolar ventilation can be calculated on the basis of CO_2 elimination from the lungs. A volume of expired gas is collected and analyzed to determine the volume of CO_2 contained. The following equation can then be utilized:

$$\dot{V}_A = \frac{\dot{V}_{CO_2}}{F_{A_{CO_2}}}$$

where

$\dot{V}_{CO_2}$ = Volume of CO_2 expired over given interval
$F_{A_{CO_2}}$ = Fraction of alveolar gas comprised by CO_2

If an end-tidal CO_2 monitor is used, a close approximation of the concentration of alveolar CO_2 is easily obtained and the equation simplified as follows:

$$\dot{V}_A = \frac{\dot{V}_{CO_2}}{\% \text{ alveolar } CO_2} \times 100$$

The same equation can be used with a substitution of the arterial P_{CO_2} for the alveolar P_{CO_2}, again presuming that arterial blood and alveolar gas are in equilibrium. The equation then becomes:

$$\dot{V}_A = \frac{\dot{V}_{CO_2}}{P_{a_{CO_2}}} \times 0.863$$

where

$P_{a_{CO_2}}$ = Arterial P_{CO_2}, which was substituted for alveolar CO_2 partial pressure

0.863 = Factor for converting from fractional concentration to partial pressure

The $\dot{V}_A$ and $\dot{V}_{CO_2}$ must both be corrected to BTPS for the equation to be valid.

Significance

Both of these methods are suitable for calculating the alveolar ventilation. The CO_2 elimination method is more accurate than the tidal volume, dead space, and rate equation when *anatomic* dead space is used in place of respiratory dead space. The difference becomes more exaggerated in cases of pronounced ventilation/blood flow inbalances. The alveolar ventilation is normally about 4 to 5 L/min with wide variations in normal individuals. The adequacy of alveolar ventilation must be ultimately determined by arterial blood gas studies.

SELECTED BIBLIOGRAPHY

Comroe, J. H., Jr.: Physiology of respiration, Chicago, 1965, Year Book Medical Publishers, Inc.

Cherniack, N. S., Lederer, D. H., Altose, M. D., and Kelson, S. G.: Occlusion pressure as a technique in evaluating respiratory control, Chest **70**:137 (supplement), 1976.

Gray, J. S., Gradius, F. S., and Carter, E. T.: Alveolar and ventilation and deadspace problem, J. Appl. Physiol. **2**:307, 1956.

Kory, R. C.: Routine measurement of respiratory rate: an expensive tribute to tradition, J.A.M.A. **165**:448, 1958.

Radford, E. P., Jr.: Ventilation standards for use in artificial respiration, J. Appl. Physiol. **10**:335, 1957.

Riley, R. L., and Cournand, A.: "Ideal" alveolar air and the analysis of ventilation-perfusion relationships in the lungs, J. Appl. Physiol. **1**:825, 1949.

Severinghaus, L. W., and Stipfel, M.: Alveolar deadspace as an index of distribution of blood flow in pulmonary capillaries, J. Appl. Physiol. **10**:335, 1957.

West, J. B.: Pulmonary pathophysiology: the essentials, Baltimore, 1977, The Williams & Wilkins Co.

West, J. B.: Respiratory physiology: the essentials, Baltimore 1974, The Williams & Wilkins Co.

CHAPTER THREE

Pulmonary mechanics tests

FORCED VITAL CAPACITY (FVC)
Description

The forced vital capacity is that volume of gas that can be expired as forcefully and rapidly as possible after maximal inspiration. FVC is always an expired volume unless specifically stated otherwise. The same maneuver performed by beginning at maximal expiration and inspiring as forcefully as possible is called forced inspiratory volume (FIV). The FVC is usually recorded in liters.

Technique

The FVC is measured by having the subject expire as forcefully and rapidly as possible into a bellows or spirometer or through a pneumotach from maximal inspiration. The volume may be read directly or from an appropriate spirographic tracing (Fig. 3-1). The volume must be corrected to BTPS.

Significance

The forced vital capacity is normally equal to the VC. The FVC may be reduced in chronic obstructive diseases, whereas the VC appears closer to normal. The forced expiration causes higher than normal transpulmonary pressures so that bronchiolar collapse, obstructive lesions, and air trapping are all exaggerated. Decreased FVC is common to restrictive diseases such as pulmonary fibrosis, as well as to obstructive processes such as emphysema and asthma.

The test's validity depends largely on patient effort and cooperation. A decreased FVC can be caused by either ob-

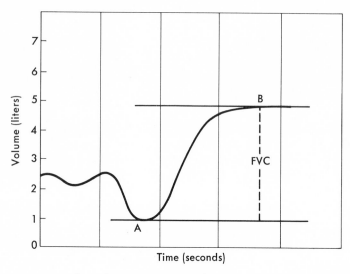

Fig. 3-1. Forced vital capacity. Typical spirogram plotting exhaled volume against time. The subject expires as rapidly and forcefully as possible from maximal inspiratory level *(A)* to maximal expiratory level *(B)*.

struction or restriction, and distinctions can often be made by comparing the FVC and the FIVC.

FORCED EXPIRATORY VOLUME (FEV$_T$)
Description

The forced expiratory volume is the volume of gas expired over a given time interval during the performance of a forced vital capacity. The interval is stated as a subscript to FEV. Those intervals in common use are FEV$_{0.5}$, FEV$_{1.0}$, FEV$_{2.0}$, and FEV$_{3.0}$. The FEV$_T$ is normally stated in liters, and T is expressed as seconds (Fig. 3-2).

Technique

The forced expiratory volume may be measured by introducing a means of timing an FVC maneuver over the de-

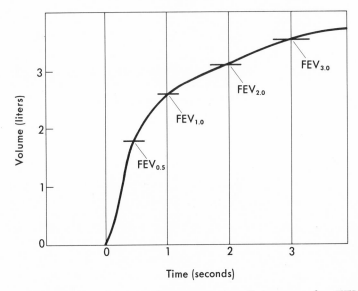

Fig. 3-2. Forced expiratory volume maneuver. Spirogram of an FEV_T maneuver, with the subject exhaling as forcefully and rapidly as possible. Marks indicate the FEV at the various intervals.

scribed intervals. Normally this is done by recording the FVC spirogram on graph paper moving at a fixed speed, so that the volume at any interval can be read from the graph. Some electronic units compute the FEV_T directly from the exhaled volume or from the instantaneous flow rate by means of appropriate transducers. Corrections to BTPS must be made.

Significance

Since the FEV_T maneuver measures a volume of gas expired over a unit of time, it is in reality a measure of flow. By assessing the flow at specific intervals, the severity of airway obstruction can be ascertained. Decreased values for FEV_T are common in both obstructive and restrictive patterns.

The validity of the test depends largely on the cooperation of the subject. The most important application of the FEV_T

is its correlation to the patient's FVC, which is normally listed as a separate test.

FORCED EXPIRATORY VOLUME/FORCED VITAL CAPACITY RATIO (FEV$_T$/FVC OR FEV$_{T\%}$)
Description

The FEV$_{T\%}$ is a statement of the FEV for a given interval expressed as a percentage of the forced vital capacity.

Technique

As described for FVC and FEV$_T$. Normally the FVC and FEV$_T$ are computed from the same test maneuver.

Significance

A normal individual can expire 50% to 60% of his FVC in 0.5 second, 75% to 85% in 1 second, 94% in 2 seconds, and 97% in 3 seconds. Patients with obstructive disease will show a reduced FEV$_{T\%}$ in most cases; patients with restrictive disease often show normal FEV$_{T\%}$, since their FVC is usually less than normal. Validity again depends on patient effort and cooperation.

FORCED EXPIRATORY FLOW$_{200-1200}$ (FEF$_{200-1200}$)
Description

The FEF$_{200-1200}$ is the *average* flow rate for the liter of gas expired after the first 200 ml during a forced expiratory volume maneuver. The same test is also termed MEFR$_{200-1200}$ (maximal expiratory flow rate). The FEF$_{200-1200}$ is usually recorded in liters per second but may be stated in liters per minute (Fig.3-3).

Technique

The FEF$_{200-1200}$ requires the same apparatus as an FEV maneuver. Normally a spirographic tracing is made, and the time interval from the 200 ml point to the 1200 ml point is divided into 1 liter to obtain the average flow rate for that interval. If the 200 and 1200 ml points are marked on the shoulder

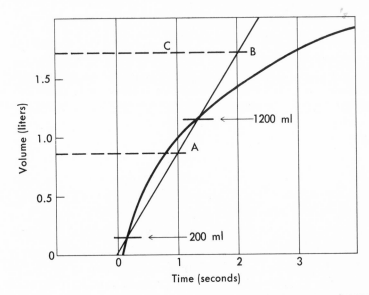

Fig. 3-3. $FEF_{200-1200}$. An FEV spirogram on which the 200 and 1200 ml points of the expiration have been marked; a line connecting these two points is extended to cross two time lines 1 second apart, points A and B. The flow rate in liters per second can be read as the vertical distance between the points of intersection (AC) and here is about 1.0 L/sec.

of the curve, a straight line connecting them may be extended so that it intersects two time lines 1 second apart on the graph paper. The flow rate may then be read as the distance between these two points of intersection (Fig. 3-3). Volumes must be corrected to BTPS.

Significance

The $FEF_{200-1200}$ measures the average flow of the early part of a forced expiration. The initial 200 ml of volume is usually expired at a slower rate because of inertia of the lung-thorax system as well as that of some types of metering systems. It is disregarded for this reason. The average rate of airflow in the initial part of a forced expiration for a healthy young man is 6 to 7 L/sec (400 L/min). The $FEF_{200-1200}$ is a good index of airflow characteristics of the larger airways, but since it is calculated from the first segment of the forced expiration, airflow slowing caused by disease of the smaller airways may be overlooked. Decreased values for $FEF_{200-1200}$ indicate a mechanical problem; obstructive disease causes a greater decrease in $FEF_{200-1200}$ than does restrictive disease. Flow rates as low as 1 L/sec (60 L/min) are not uncommon in obstructive patterns. $FEF_{200-1200}$ decreases significantly with age and is normally lower in women than in men. (See the Appendix.) The nature of the mechanical problem in decreased flow rates is sometimes clarified by measuring the average *inspiratory* flow rate, for the same part of the FIV. Healthy young men can normally attain rates of 5 L/sec (300 L/min) on inspiration. This test is usually designated $FIF_{200-1200}$ (forced inspiratory flow) or $MIFR_{200-1200}$. The validity of the test depends on subject cooperation and effort.

FORCED EXPIRATORY FLOW$_{25\%-75\%}$ ($FEF_{25\%-75\%}$)
Description

The $FEF_{25\%-75\%}$ is the average rate of flow during the middle half of a forced expiratory volume. It is recorded in liters per second or liters per minute. The same test is also designated maximum midexpiratory flow rate (MMFR).

Technique

The $FEF_{25\%-75\%}$ requires the same apparatus as an FEV maneuver. The length of time required for the subject to expire 50% of his vital capacity (forced) after he has exhaled the initial 25% of his FVC is divided into 50% of his FVC. Normally a spirogram is used, with 25% and 75% points marked on the curve (Fig. 3-4). A straight line connecting these points is extended to intersect two time lines 1 second apart, and the flow rate can be read directly as the distance between the points of intersection. The $FEF_{25\%-75\%}$ can be computed electronically, but may be in error depending on the triggering mechanism of the particular instrument. Volumes must be corrected to BTPS.

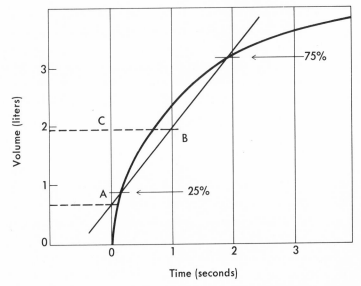

Fig. 3-4. FEF$_{25\%-75\%}$. An FEV spirogram on which the 25% and 75% points of expiration have been marked; these points are determined by multiplying the FVC by 0.25 and 0.75, respectively. A line connecting these points is extended to intersect two time lines 1 second apart, points *A* and *B*. The flow rate in liters per second can be read as the vertical distance between the points of intersection *(AC)*—in this case a little over 1 L/sec.

Significance

The FEF$_{25\%-75\%}$, like the FEF$_{200-1200}$, measures the average flow rate over a given interval (volume) but is based on a segment of the FVC that includes more than the initial part of the breath. It is normally somewhat slower than the FEF$_{200-1200}$, the values for healthy young men averaging 4.7 L/sec (282 L/min). The FEF$_{25\%-75\%}$ is indicative of the status of the medium-sized airways. Decreased flow rates are common in the early stages of obstructive disease, more so than in restrictive disease. Flows as low as 0.3 L/sec (20 L/min) may occur in severe cases of obstruction, such as advanced emphysema. The FEF$_{25\%-75\%}$ values also decrease with age. The test depends on voluntary effort but is more reproducible than the $FEF_{200-1200}$. There is little evidence that $FEF_{25\%-75\%}$ is more reliable than other flow measurements commonly used in assessing obstructive ventilatory impairments, although it seems to be more commonly used. Fig. 3-5 shows typical abnormal spirograms for obstructive and restrictive patterns.

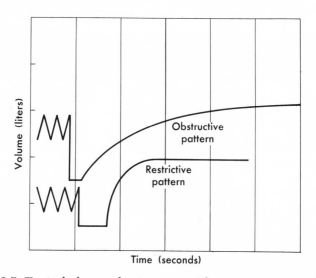

Fig. 3-5. Typical abnormal spirograms. *Obstructive pattern* shows decreased FVC (less than 2.0 L) as well as expiratory airflow slowing; volume expired in 1 sec is much less than 75% of FVC (FEV_1/FVC). $FEF_{25\%-75\%}$, if calculated as described in the text, would derive values much lower than normal. *Restrictive pattern* also shows a reduced FVC, approximately equal to that in the obstructive pattern, but FEV_1/FVC is *increased;* that is, almost all of the FVC is expired in the first second. $FEF_{25\%-75\%}$ is also close to expected normal values. FVC alone cannot be used to distinguish obstructive from restrictive disease patterns; flow rates are typically decreased in obstructive lung disease and are only decreased significantly in pure restrictive disease when lung volumes are greatly reduced. FEV_1/FVC ratios should always be correlated to the actual measured values obtained for FEV_1 and FVC to help ascertain the nature of the lesion.

PEAK FLOW (PEFR)
Description

The peak flow is the maximum flow rate attainable at any time during a forced expiratory volume. It is recorded in liters per second or liters per minute.

Technique

The peak flow can be measured by drawing a tangent to the "steepest" part of an FVC spirogram. The tracing should be made with the pen or paper moving at the fastest possible

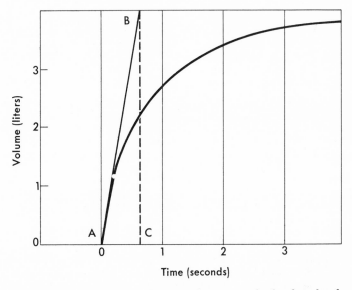

Fig. 3-6. Peak flow tangent. FEV spirogram on which a line has been drawn tangent to the steepest part of the curve, line *AB*. Normally the steepest part of the curve is near the very beginning. In this case the tangent has a slope such that it does not intersect the two closest time lines, 1 second apart. The flow rate can be computed by dividing the volume *(BC)* by the time interval *(AC)*, of 4 L/0.67 sec. The peak flow in this instance then is approximately 6 L/sec. This method is somewhat less than precise, especially in normal individuals, whose peak flows often exceed 10 L/sec. The pneumotach offers better results, especially at high flows. (See text.)

speed. The tangent may be extended to intersect two time lines and the flow read directly as the distance between the points of intersection for that interval (Fig. 3-6). Peak flow may be measured accurately by means of a pneumotachometer, or electronic pneumotachometer, which uses a transducer to convert flow or pressure to an electrical output that is displayed on a meter. (See Chapter 8.) Temperature corrections must be made.

Significance

Peak flows as computed by the first method just given are of doubtful accuracy, especially in normal subjects. The peak flow attainable in healthy young men may exceed 10 L/sec (600 L/min). Even when measured by the pneumotachometer, peak flow measurements are of limited value. Patients with obstructive disease may develop an initially high flow rate before airway closing occurs. Decreased peak flow is indicative of a mechanical problem but is largely nonspecific. The test, of course, depends on subject effort.

MAXIMUM VOLUNTARY VENTILATION (MVV)
Description

Maximal voluntary ventilation is the largest volume that can be breathed per minute by voluntary effort. It is recorded in liters per minute.

Technique

The maximum voluntary ventilation is measured by having the subject breathe as deeply and rapidly as possible. He should set his own rate and move more than his tidal volume but less than his vital capacity on each breath. The test is conducted for a specific interval (10, 12, or 15 seconds). The volume expired (or inspired) may be measured in a bellows or spirometer. The volume may be read directly or from an appropriate spirogram (Fig. 3-7). The actual values are extrapolated from 10, 12, or 15 seconds to 1 minute and the result recorded as a flow rate, in liters per minute. The volumes must be corrected to BTPS.

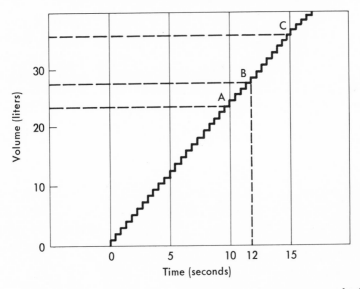

Fig. 3-7. Maximum voluntary ventilation. MVV spirogram on which totalized volume is plotted against time. Since the MVV is stated as a flow rate in liters per minute, the values for 10, 12, and 15 seconds must be extrapolated to 1 minute. Hence $MVV_{10} \times 6 = MVV$ (L/min), $MVV_{12} \times 5 = MVV$ (L/min), $MVV_{15} \times 4 = MVV$ (L/min). Normal subjects will maintain the same MVV flow rate at 10, 12, and 15 seconds. Patients with pulmonary disease will show decreased absolute values, and oftentimes the MVV_{12} and MVV_{15} will be significantly less than the MVV_{10} because of fatigue of the respiratory muscles, increased work of breathing, etc.

Significance

Maximal voluntary ventilation measures the status of the respiratory muscles, the compliance of the lung-thorax system, and the resistance offered by the airways and tissues. Normal values vary by as much as 30% from the mean, so that only large reductions in MVV are truly significant. Healthy young adults (men) average 170 L/min. Values are lower in healthy women and decrease with age in both men and women. MVV is decreased greatly in patients with moderate to severe obstructive disease. The maneuver exaggerates air trapping and exertion of the respiratory muscles. MVV may be within normal limits even in some patients with restrictive pulmonary disease, since limitation of thoracic expansion does not in most cases impede the respiratory muscles. The MVV and vital capacity of an individual are sometimes expressed as a ratio $\left(\dfrac{\% \text{ of predicted MVV}}{\% \text{ of predicted VC}}\right)$ called the *air velocity index*, but this is of little value apart from the absolute values for MVV and VC. The MVV maneuver depends largely on patient effort.

COMPLIANCE (C)
Description

Compliance is the volume change per unit of pressure change for the lungs (C_L), the thorax (C_T), or the lungs-thorax system (C_{LT}). The compliance for all three is recorded in liters per centimeter of water.

Technique

The compliance of the lungs-thorax system (C_{LT}) may be measured as a unit, or the compliance of the lungs alone (C_L) determined and the compliance of the thorax calculated by subtraction.

The C_{LT} is measured by having a subject in a sealed chamber inspire measured volumes by reducing the "atmospheric" pressure as in an "iron lung"; a volume pressure curve is then plotted. The subject may likewise be intubated with an endotracheal tube and pressure changes at various volumes above the end-expiratory level plotted to obtain a pressure-volume curve. This technique requires that the subject be anesthetized. Or a subject may be allowed to inspire known volumes from a spirometer and pressure changes measured by means of a nasal plug in one nostril connected to a manometer. The subject must be instructed to relax all respiratory muscles so that the nasal pressure approximates alveolar pressure.

Measurement of pulmonary compliance (C_L) is accomplished by passing a balloon catheter into the esophagus at midthorax level and connecting it to a manometer. Serial pressure changes can be recorded at various volumes and plotted (Fig. 3-8). All these measurements must be made under static conditions, with no airflow. Thoracic compliance (C_T) can be derived if total and pulmonary compliances are known:

$$\frac{1}{C_{LT}} - \frac{1}{C_L} = \frac{1}{C_T}$$

Significance

Measurements of compliance determine the elasticity of the lungs, the thorax, and the combination of the two. The av-

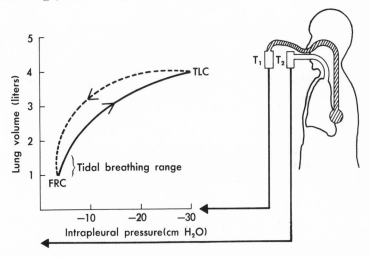

Fig. 3-8. Measurement of pulmonary compliance (esophageal balloon technique). Determination of pulmonary compliance (C_L) requires measurement of intrapleural pressure at various lung volumes. Transducer T_1 is connected to an esophageal balloon containing a small amount of air and monitors changes in intrapleural pressure (ΔP). Transducer T_2 is actually a flow transducer (pneumotach) and is used to measure inspired or expired gas volumes (ΔV). Static pulmonary compliance is the slope of the line defined by:

$$\frac{\Delta V \text{ (liters)}}{\Delta P \text{ (cm } H_2O)}$$

and is normally recorded from the tidal breathing range. Pulmonary compliance varies with the lung volume history, as illustrated by the steeper *expiratory* pressure-volume curve. Compliance measurements are often performed with the subject in the body plethysmograph to facilitate determination of absolute lung volumes.

erage *pulmonary* compliance in a normal adult is 0.2 L/cm H_2O. The *thoracic* compliance is also 0.2 L/cm H_2O. In series, the *total* compliance is:

$$\frac{1}{C_L} + \frac{1}{C_T} = \frac{1}{C_{LT}}$$

or

$$\frac{1}{0.2} + \frac{1}{0.2} = 0.1 \text{ L/cm } H_2O$$

The total compliance is less than either of its two components because of the counterbalancing forces of the lungs and the thorax.

Pulmonary compliance varies with the volume of the lungs at the end-expiratory level (FRC). To compare the compliance of diseased lungs with that of normal lungs, the FRC in each case should be known. This is often stated as the compliance/FRC ratio. The C_{LT}/FRC ratio for adults ranges from 0.05 to 0.06. Pulmonary compliance is normally decreased in pulmonary edema or congestion, atelectasis, pneumonia, loss of surfactant, and restrictive diseases such as pulmonary fibrosis. These decreases of course may in many cases be caused by reduction of FRC. Emphysema is normally accompanied by an increase in compliance, since less pressure is required to maintain the FRC in the lungs. However, thoracic compliance may be decreased in obstructive diseases because of chronic hyperinflation; hence total compliance may appear normal. Total compliance may be decreased as a result of thoracic disease such as kyphoscoliosis or because of abdominal disorders such as obesity.

A special application of the determination of compliance is the measurement of lung compliance at various breathing frequencies. Obstructive disease processes in airways smaller than 2 mm in diameter cause different regions of the lungs to ventilate asynchronously. This phenomenon can be detected by measurement of compliance at rapid breathing rates, usually 80 to 100 per minute. Compliance measured during breathing is called dynamic compliance (Cdyn). Normal sub-

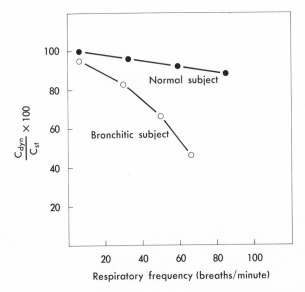

Fig. 3-9. Frequency dependence of compliance. Dynamic compliance (Cdyn) as a percentage of static compliance (Cst) for a normal subject (·---) and a bronchitic subject (o-o-o-) is plotted at increasing respiratory frequencies. Increased resistance in small airways (< 2 mm) causes uneven distribution of gas, with most gas going to those lung units with normal resistance. At times of zero gas flow at the mouth, gas is still moving within the lung from one region to another (the Pendelluft phenomenon). Since some regions are out of phase with others, gas distribution becomes more uneven as breathing frequency increases and causes a fall in the ratio of dynamic to static compliance.

jects exhibit similar values for compliance under both static (Cst) and dynamic conditions. The frequency dependence of compliance is expressed as the ratio of Cdyn/Cst × 100. Values of less than 80% for this ratio are consistent with small airway obstruction. Frequency dependence is a very sensitive indicator of obstruction in smaller airways and may be present in persons with asthma and bronchitis in whom conventional tests such as FEV_1, $FEF_{25\%-75\%}$, and R_{aw} are within normal limits (Fig. 3-9).

AIRWAY RESISTANCE (R_{aw}) AND CONDUCTANCE (G_{aw})

Description

Airway resistance (R_{aw}) is the pressure difference required for a unit flow change. This pressure difference is created by the friction of flowing molecules coming in contact with the conducting airways. Airway resistance is recorded in centimeters of water per liter per second. Airway conductance (G_{aw}) is the flow generated per unit of pressure drop in the airway. It is the reciprocal of R_{aw} and is recorded in liters per second per centimeter of water.

Technique

Airway resistance (R_{aw}) is the ratio of alveolar pressure (Pa) to airflow ($\dot{V}$). Gas flow can be measured easily with a pneumotachograph, and alveolar pressure is measured with a body plethysmograph (Fig. 3-10). For gas to flow into the lungs (inspiration), alveolar pressure must fall below atmospheric pressure; the opposite occurs during expiration. Since the total volume of gas in the lungs and plethysmograph remains constant, the changes in alveolar pressure are reflected by reciprocal changes in the plethysmograph. (Pressures are monitored by sensitive pressure transducers at the mouth and in the plethysmograph, and flow is measured with a heated pneumotach). Changes in airflow are plotted simultaneously against plethysmographic pressure changes (which are proportional to alveolar pressure changes) on a storage oscilloscope.

The slope of this line is $\dot{V}/P_P$, where $\dot{V}$ is airflow and P_P is the plethysmograph pressure. Immediately after this measurement, an electronic shutter at the mouthpiece is closed and changes in plethysmograph pressure are plotted against the airway pressure at the mouth. Since there is no airflow into or out of the lungs, the mouth pressure approximates alveolar pressure. The slope of this line is P_A/P_P, where P_A equals alveolar pressure. This step serves to calibrate changes in alveolar pressure to changes in plethysmograph pressure for each subject.

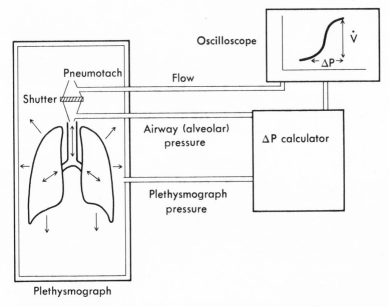

Fig. 3-10. Measurement of airway resistance. Diagrammatic representation of the measurement of airway resistance by the body plethysmograph method:

$$\text{Airway resistance} = \frac{\text{Atmospheric pressure} - \text{Alveolar pressure}}{\text{Flow}}$$

Flow $(\dot{V})$ is measured directly by means of the pneumotach. The pressure differential between the chamber and the alveoli is measured thus: plethysmograph pressure is monitored by means of a sensitive manometer in the chamber; alveolar pressure is measured as airway pressure during intervals when no gas flow is occurring. A shutter occludes the airway momentarily, usually at end-expiration, and a manometer monitors the falling pressure. The pressure differential is calculated and delivered to an appropriate display device (X-Y recorder, oscilloscope).

The airway resistance, R_{aw}, is then calculated by taking the ratio for these two slopes:

$$R_{aw} = \frac{P_A/P_P}{\dot{V}/P_P}$$

where

   $\dot{V}$ = Airflow

   P_A = Alveolar pressure

   P_P = Plethysmographic pressure, which is the same measured with the shutter opened and closed

These measurements are made with the subject panting with an open glottis. Panting eliminates a number of artifacts from the tracing and allows measurements to be made at or near FRC. Corrections for the resistance of the mouthpiece and flowmeter are made. Conductance (G_{aw}) can be simply calculated as the reciprocal of R_{aw}. Lung volumes are normally measured by the plethysmograph method (see p. 10) immediately after R_{aw} is measured, thus allowing the calculation of specific conductance (SG_{aw}) and specific resistance (SR_{aw}).

Significance

Normal values of airway resistance in adult subjects, panting and using a plethysmograph, range from 0.6 to 2.4 cm $H_2O/L/sec$. Measurements are normally standardized at a flow rate of 0.5 L/sec.

Airway resistance is increased in asthma during an acute episode by as much as three times the normal values. Resistance is increased in emphysema because of airway narrowing and collapse in some of the larger airways as well as the more distal passages. Other obstructive diseases, such as bronchitis, cause increases in airway resistance proportionate to the degree of obstruction.

Measurement of airway resistance is often useful in distinguishing between restrictive and obstructive diseases. The test is objective insofar as the patient cannot influence results by degree of effort. Because resistance is decreased by increased lung volume, it is often advantageous to ascertain the FRC at the time of the resistance measurement. To use conductance or resistance for comparative study, these values are often expressed per unit of lung volume. By dividing R_{aw} or G_{aw} by the lung volume at which the measurement was made, the specific resistance and conductance are obtained and are expressed as R_{aw}/V_L and G_{aw}/V_L, respectively. These terms are sometimes referred to as SR_{aw} and SG_{aw}. This can be done easily with the body plethysmograph (Chapter 1). In addition to resistance caused by airflow through the conducting tubes, some of the total pulmonary resistance results from the friction caused by displacement of the lungs, rib cage, and diaphragm. Normally, this "tissue" resistance is only about one fifth of the total resistance, and therefore pulmonary resistance is approximately 20% greater than the measured airway resistance.

FLOW-VOLUME CURVES (MEFV)
Description

The flow-volume curve is a graphic analysis of the flow generated during a foraced expiratory volume maneuver followed by a forced inspiratory volume maneuver, versus the volume expired (Fig. 3-11). The flow is usually recorded in liters per second and the volume in liters. The maximal expiratory flow-volume (MEFV) curve or tracing delineates the expiratory portion of the curve in particular without reference to the inspiratory loop.

Technique

The subject performs an FEV maneuver followed by an FIV maneuver. The expired volume is plotted on the abscissa and the amount of flow generated on the ordinate. This type of spirogram must be done with a recorder capable of plotting flow and volume from their respective electrical inputs. (See Fig. 8-6). From the graph the peak inspiratory and expiratory flows can be read, as well as the FVC. The instantaneous flow at any lung volume can be read directly from the MEFV tracing. The flow at 50% and 25% of the VC are commonly reported as the $\dot{V}_{max\ 50}$ and $\dot{V}_{max\ 25}$, respectively. If an automatic timer is available on the graphing device, the FEV_T can also be determined for whatever intervals are measured.

Significance

Predicted values for FEV_T (if time marks are incorporated into the MEFV tracing) and for the FVC are the same as for conventional volume-time curves. Significant decreases in

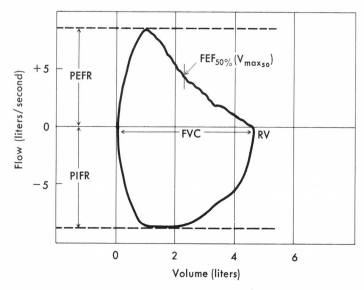

Fig. 3-11. Flow-volume loop. Flow-volume spirogram in which an FEV and an FIV maneuver are recorded in succession. Flow rate is plotted on the vertical axis and volume on the horizontal axis. Peak flows for inspiration and expiration can be read directly, as can the FVC. The instantaneous flow rate at a particular point in the FVC can be measured directly. Recorders that are capable of interjecting time marks, or "tics," in the tracing allow the FEV_T to be read directly as well. Phenomena such as airway collapse show up as abrupt changes in the flow rate.

either flow or volume (obstructive or restrictive processes) are available in single graphic display to aid in differentiating specific lesions. The shape of the expiratory curve of the MEFV tracing from about 75% of TLC down to RV is largely independent of patient effort, flow being determined mainly by the elastic recoil properties of the lungs. In normal subjects, flow ($\dot{V}_{max}$) decreases linearly with volume over most of the VC range, so that the curve has "straight line" appearance (Fig. 3-11). In patients with obstructive lung disease, flow is decreased particularly at lower lung volumes and the inde-

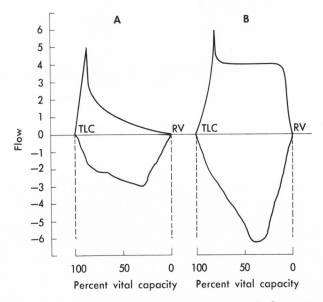

Fig. 3-12. Flow volume curves characteristic of obstruction. **A,** MEFV curve shows decreased maximal flow rates at almost all lung volumes consistent with *small airway obstruction.* The typical "scooped out" appearance of the expiratory limb is common to diseases affecting the small airways, such as asthma and emphysema. The FVC may be normal or decreased; peak expiratory flow may be decreased only slightly. **B,** MEFV curve shows *variable obstruction to flow,* consistent with an intrathoracic obstruction of a larger airway, such as tracheal or bronchial tumor. The characteristic appearance is the "squared off" expiratory limb. The FVC again may be normal or decreased; peak flow may also be close to normal; inspiratory flow curve may be completely normal.

pendent segment of the flow volume curve takes on a curvilinear or "scooped out" appearance (Fig. 3-12). Values for $\dot{V}_{max\ 50}$ and $\dot{V}_{max\ 25}$ are characteristically decreased. Decreases in $\dot{V}_{max\ 50}$ correlate well with the $FEF_{25\%-75\%}$ in subjects with obstructive lung disease.

Obstruction of the upper airway, trachea, and mainstem bronchi show characteristic limitations to expiratory flow, and thus the flow-volume curve is useful in diagnosing these particular lesions (Fig. 3-12).

Restrictive processes may show relatively normal peak expiratory flows and linear decrease in flow versus lung volume, but the lung volume itself is decreased. Moderate to severe restriction demonstrates equally reduced flows at all lung volumes and may appear as a "miniature" of the normal MEFV curve.

Before and after bronchodilator MEFV curves can be superimposed to facilitate measurement of relative increases in flow at each lung volume. Similarly, tidal breathing curves and MVV curves can be superimposed on the flow-volume curve (inspiratory and expiratory curves) to evaluate ventilatory reserves by comparing the areas bounded by each of the curves. Subjects with severe chronic obstructive lung disease often generate flow-volume curves of only slightly greater dimensions than their tidal breathing curves.

VOLUME OF ISOFLOW (Viso$\dot{V}$)
Description

The volume of isoflow (Viso$\dot{V}$) is that part of the VC remaining in the lungs at which gas flow becomes independent of gas density and is determined by superimposing MEFV curves recorded with the subject breathing air and a mixture of 80% helium and 20% oxygen (Fig. 3-13). The volume of isoflow is recorded as a percentage of the FVC.

Technique

Maximal expiratory flow-volume (MEFV) curves are obtained in subjects after breathing air. The MEFV maneuver is repeated with the subject breathing the He-O_2 mixture. The subject may either breathe the mixture for 10 minutes or take three slow vital capacity breaths of the mixture before performing the maneuver; both techniques yield results that do not differ significantly. The He-O_2 mixture and air curves are then superimposed and matched at residual volume if the FVC values are different. The point at which the curves meet determines that part of the FVC that remains in the lungs

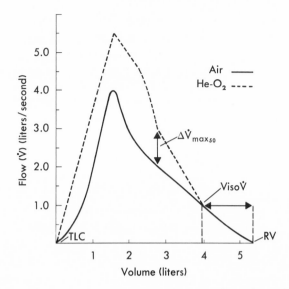

Fig. 3-13. Helium-oxygen–air MEFV curves. The subject performs two MEFV maneuvers; the first is a simple MEFV maneuver breathing air; the second MEFV maneuver is performed after the subject has breathed a mixture of 80% He and 20% O_2 for several minutes or for several vital capacity breaths. The two curves are then superimposed by matching at residual volume (RV). The $\dot{V}_{max50}$ (or $\dot{V}_{max}$ at any other lung volume) can then be read directly from the tracing. Decreases in the $\dot{V}_{max50}$ are consistent with diseases causing increased resistance in the small airways (< 2 mm), but there is apparently little change with loss of elastic recoil. The point at which both curves converge is the volume of isoflow (Viso$\dot{V}$). At this lung volume, maximum expiratory flow becomes independent of the gas density of the expirate. Diseases that compromise the small airways, either by increased resistance or loss of elastic recoil, tend to increase the volume of isoflow, so that the curves converge earlier during the expiratory maneuver.

when gas flow becomes identical after breathing air and the He-O_2 mixture (Fig. 3-13). This lung volume is known as the isoflow volume and is expressed as a percentage of the FVC. From the same tracing, the increase in maximal flow at 50% of the vital capacity ($\dot{V}_{max\ 50}$) can be determined. Since flow in larger airways depends on gas density, the amount of increase in $\dot{V}_{max\ 50}$ while breathing the He-O_2 mixture is relatively specific for changes in airway caliber. The increase in $\dot{V}_{max\ 50}$ while breathing the He-O_2 mixture is expressed as a percentage of the $\dot{V}_{max\ 50}$ while breathing air and is called the $\Delta\dot{V}_{max\ 50}$:

$$\Delta\dot{V}_{max\ 50} = \frac{\dot{V}_{max\ 50_{He}} - \dot{V}_{max\ 50_{air}}}{\dot{V}_{max\ 50_{air}}} \times 100$$

Significance

Normal values for Viso$\dot{V}$ as a percentage of the FVC appear to be in the range of 10% to 20% for subjects 20 to 50 years of age.

An increase in the volume of isoflow above the normal level is consistent with obstruction of small airways. During forced expiration in normal subjects, the site of flow limitation is in the large airways until low lung volumes are reached. Breathing a gas of low density improves flow in these larger airways, but as flow limitation shifts to the smaller airways (less than 2 mm) toward the end of a forced expiration, resistance is determined by laminar airflow and is independent of gas density. At this point the He-O_2 mixture and air curves converge. Therefore, in diseases of the small airways in which there is increased resistance (asthma) or in which there is a loss of elastic recoil (emphysema), the site of flow limitation is located in the smaller airways at a higher lung volume and Viso$\dot{V}$ is increased.

The increase in $\Delta\dot{V}_{max\ 50}$ is reduced in diseases that cause increased resistance, although loss of elastic recoil does not appear to influence $\Delta\dot{V}_{max\ 50}$. Thus $\Delta\dot{V}_{max\ 50}$ is relatively specific for changes in the caliber of small airways.

The volume of isoflow is one of the most sensitive tests of small airway obstruction. It is relatively simple to perform and, in combination with measurement of the $\Delta\dot{V}_{max\ 50}$, may be helpful in differentiating large and small airway disease and determining whether the loss of elastic recoil or increased resistance is the causative factor.

SELECTED BIBLIOGRAPHY

Bates, D. V., Macklem, P. T., and Christie, R. V.: Respiratory function in disease, ed. 2, Philadelphia, 1971, W. B. Saunders Co.

Bode, F. R., Dosman, J., Martin, R. R., Macklem, P. T.: Reversibility of pulmonary function abnormalities in smokers, Am. J. Med. **59**:43, 1975.

Comroe, J. H., Jr.: Physiology of respiration, Chicago, 1965, Year Book Medical Publishers, Inc.

Comroe, J. H., Jr., Forster, R. E., II, Dubois, A. B., Briscoe, W. H., and Carlsen, E.: The lung: clinical physiology and pulmonary function tests, ed. 2, Chicago, 1962, Year Book Medical Publishers, Inc.

Despas, P. J., Leroux, M., and Macklem, P. T.: Site of airway obstruction in asthma as determined by measuring flow breathing air and a helium-oxygen mixture, J. Clin. Invest. **51**:3235, 1972.

Dosman, J., Bode, F., Urbanetti, J., Martin, R., and Macklem, P. T.: The use of a helium-oxygen mixture during maximum expiratory flow to demonstrate obstruction in small airways in smokers, J. Clin. Invest. **55**:1090, 1975.

Dubois, A. B., Botelho, S. V., and Comroe, J. H., Jr.: A new method for measuring airway resistance in man using a body plethysmograph: values in normal subjects and in patients with respiratory disease, J. Clin. Invest. **35**:327, 1956.

Fry, D. L., and Hyatt, R. E.: Pulmonary mechanics: a unified analysis of the relationship between pressure, volume, and gas flow in the lungs of normal and diseased human subjects, Am. J. Med. **292**:672, 1960.

Gelb, A. F., and Klein, E.: The volume of isoflow and increase in maximal flow at 50 percent of forced vital capacity during helium-oxygen breathing as tests of small airway dysfunction, Chest **71**:396, 1977.

Gelb, A. F., Maloney, P. A., Klein, E., and Aronstam, P. S.: Sensitivity of volume of isoflow in the detection of mild airway obstruction, Am. Rev. Respir. Dis. **112**:401, 1975.

Hogg, J. C., Macklem, P. T., and Thurlbeck, W. M.: Site and nature of airway obstruction in chronic obstructive lung disease, N. Engl. J. Med. **278**:1355, 1968.

Hyatt, R. E.: Dynamic lung volumes. In Fenn, W. O., and Rahn, H., editors: Handbook of physiology—respiration II, Washington, D.C., 1965, American Physiological Society, pp. 1381-1397.

Hyatt, R. E., and Black, L. F.: The flow-volume curve, Am. Rev. Respir. Dis. **107**:191, 1973.

Kory, R. C., Callahan, R., Boren, H. G., and Syner, J. C.: The Veterans Administration—Army Cooperative Study of Pulmonary Function. I. Clinical spirometry in normal men, Am. J. Med. **30**:243, 1961.

Leuallen, E. C., and Fowler, W. S.: Maximal midexpiratory flow, Am. Rev. Tuberculosis **72**:783, 1955.

Marshall, R.: Objective tests of respiratory mechanics. In Fenn, W. O., and Rahn, H., editors: Handbook of physiology—respiration II, Washington, D.C., 1965, American Physiological Society, pp. 1399-1410.

McNeill, R. S., Malcolm, G. D., and Brown, W. R.: Comparison of expiratory and inspiratory flow rates in health and in chronic pulmonary disease, Thorax **14**:225, 1959.

Morris, J. F., Koski, A., and Johnson, L. C.: Spirometric standards for healthy non-smoking adults, Am. Rev. Respir. Dis. **107**:57, 1971.

Woolcock, A. J., Vincent, N. J., and Macklem, P. T.: Frequency dependence of compliance as a test for obstruction in the small airways, J. Clin. Invest. **48**:1099, 1969.

CHAPTER FOUR

Gas distribution tests

SINGLE-BREATH NITROGEN ELIMINATION (SBN₂), CLOSING VOLUME (CV), AND CLOSING CAPACITY (CC)

Description

The single-breath $\%N_2$ test measures the increase in the concentration of N_2 in the 500 ml of gas exhaled after the first 750 ml of a single breath of 100% oxygen. The single-breath nitrogen concentration is recorded as a percentage.

The closing volume is the lung volume at which airway closure begins. Closing volume is expressed as a percentage of the vital capacity. Closing capacity is the sum of the closing volume and residual volume (RV) (see Chapter 1) and is expressed as a percentage of the total lung capacity.

Technique

The subject expires to residual volume, then inhales a single breath of 100% O_2. Without holding his breath, the subject expires slowly and evenly into a spirometer through an N_2 analyzer that rapidly monitors the N_2 concentration of the expired gas. Expired volume, as measured by the spirometer, is plotted against N_2 concentration on a suitable graph (Fig. 4-1). The curves can be divided into four phases: Phase I is extreme upper airway gas consisting of 100% O_2; Phase II is mixed dead space gas in which the relative concentrations of O_2 and N_2 change abruptly as the dead space volume is expired; Phase III is a plateau caused by the exhalation of alveolar gas, whose relative O_2 and N_2 concentrations change slowly and evenly; Phase IV is noted by an abrupt increase in the concentration of N_2 tht continues until residual volume is reached.

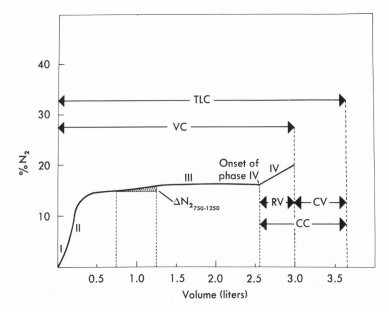

Fig. 4-1. Single-breath nitrogen elimination (SBN$_2$). Plot of the rise in nitrogen concentration on expiration following a single vital capacity breath of pure O$_2$. The curve is divided into four parts or phases. Phase I is the extreme beginning of the expiration when only pure O$_2$ is being exhaled. Phase II shows an abrupt rise in N$_2$ concentration as mixed bronchial and alveolar air is expired. Phase III is the alveolar gas plateau, and nitrogen concentration changes only slightly as long as ventilation is uniformly distributed. Phase IV is an abrupt increase in N$_2$ concentration as basal airways close and a larger proportion of gas comes from the nitrogen-rich lung apices. Several useful parameters are derived from the SBN$_2$ tracing. Anatomic dead space can be calculated (see Chapter 2). The $\Delta N_{2_{750-1250}}$ and slope of Phase III are indices of the evenness of ventilation distribution. Closing volume can be read directly from the onset of Phase IV until RV is reached; vital capacity can also be read directly. RV, TLC, and CC can be calculated if the area under the curve is determined either by planimetry or electronic integration. (See text.)

The initial 750 ml of expired gas contain the dead space volume of Phases I and II and is disregarded. The difference in N_2 concentration between the 750 ml and 1250 ml points is called the delta $N_2(\Delta N_{2_{750-1250}})$. The volume expired after the onset of Phase IV is called the closing volume (CV). The closing volume may be added to the residual volume, if determined, and expressed as the closing capacity (CC). Closing volume is normally recorded as a percentage of the vital capacity:

$$CV/VC \times 100$$

Closing capacity is recorded as a percentage of the total lung capacity:

$$CC/TLC \times 100$$

Total lung capacity can be determined from the SBN_2 test by using a dilution equation to calculate RV and adding it to the measured vital capacity. Residual volume is calculated as follows:

$$RV = VC \times \frac{F_{\bar{E}N_2}}{F_{AN_2} - F_{\bar{E}N_2}}$$

where

$F_{\bar{E}N_2}$ = Mean expired N_2 concentration determined by planimetry or electronic integration of the area under the curve

F_{AN_2} = N_2 concentration in the lungs at the beginning of inspiration, approximately 0.75 to 0.79

This method is accurate only in subjects without significant obstructive disease or dead space producing disease.

Significance

$\Delta N_{2_{750-1250}}$. The normal $\Delta N_{2_{750-1250}}$ is 1.5% or less for healthy young adults and slightly higher for healthy older adults (approximately 3%). Increases in $\Delta N_{2_{750-1250}}$s are found in diseases characterized by uneven gas distribution during inspiration and unequal flow rates during expiration. In patients with severe emphysema, $\Delta N_{2_{750-1250}}$ may exceed 10%. A best-fit line drawn through the Phase III segment of the tracing from about 30% of the vital capacity to the onset of Phase IV is used to determine the slope of Phase III. This slope is used as an index of gas distribution, in a manner similar to the $\Delta N_{2_{750-1250}}$. Very slow expiratory flow rates may cause oscillations in the tracing of Phase III, making the accurate measurement of the $\Delta N_{2_{750-1250}}$ difficult. These oscillations are attributed to changes in alveolar N_2 concentrations as blood pulses through the pulmonary capillaries during cardiac systole. Increasing the expiratory flow rate eliminates this common artifact.

CV and CC. Phase IV of the SBN_2 test can be explained by the fact that after a maximal expiration there is proportionately more residual volume gas at the apices of the lungs than at the bases, and when a test gas is inspired the apices receive the gas occupying the subject's dead space, with the test gas then going preferentially to the bases of the lungs. Gas concentrations in the lung become widely different since the apices contain residual volume gas plus dead space gas (largely nitrogen), while the bases contain predominately test gas (oxygen in this case). Dynamic compression of the airways during the subsequent exhalation causes airways to close as lung volume approaches RV. Basilar airways close first because of gravity and the weight of the lung in upright subjects. As the composition of gas switches from test gas to higher concentrations of N_2, Phase IV begins.

Closing volume and closing capacity indicate the lung volume at which airway closure begins and are thus indices of the status of the small airways. Closing volume and closing capacity may be increased (earlier onset of airway closure) with increase in age, in restrictive processes in which the FRC becomes less than CV, in smokers and other subjects with early obstructive disease of small airways, and in congestive heart failure when the caliber of the small airways is compromised.

Subjects with moderate to severe obstructive disease may

display no sharp demarcation between Phase III and Phase IV of the SBN_2 because of grossly uneven distribution of gas in the lungs with little difference in gas composition between apices and bases.

Closing volume and closing capacity measurements may be in error if the subject does not perform a true vital capacity maneuver. Vital capacity during the CV determination should not differ more than 5% from the subject's reproducible VC. Expiratory flow should be maintained between 0.3 and 0.5 L/sec.

To calculate normal values for CV and CC according to age and sex, see the Appendix.

NITROGEN WASHOUT TEST (7-MINUTE)
Description

The N_2 washout test measures the concentration of N_2 in alveolar gas at the end of 7 minutes of 100% O_2 breathing. The N_2 washout test value is recorded as a percentage of nitrogen.

Technique

The simplest method of calculating the degree of N_2 washout in the lungs is by having the subject breathe pure O_2 for 7 minutes, then measuring the N_2 concentration of a sample of alveolar gas collected at the end of a forced expiration. The evenness of ventilation determines whether practically all the N_2 has been washed out by O_2.

A test of more quantitative value is that in which the dilution of N_2 by oxygen is graphed or displayed for each breath by means of rapid analysis of expired gas. Normally the $\%N_2$ is plotted against the expired volume or number of breaths. The typical washout curve is an exponential, or J-shaped, curve, which becomes a straight line when the $\%N_2$ is graphed on semilog paper (Fig. 4-2).

Significance

The normal value for the concentration of N_2 in alveolar gas after 7 minutes of O_2 breathing is less than 2.5%. The ac-

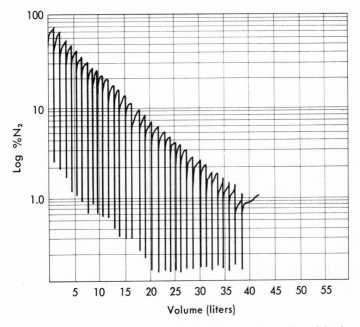

Fig. 4-2. Nitrogen washout (7-minute). Illustrated is a plot of the logarithm of the nitrogen concentration versus expired volume. The elimination of nitrogen from the lungs by O_2 breathing occurs exponentially. A single-chambered lung being washed out in this fashion would produce a J-shaped curve; however, when the $\%N_2$ is plotted on semilog paper, the result is a straight line. Normal lungs produce an approximately straight line; lungs with deranged distribution tend to show a fast washout initially and progressive slowing as the test proceeds. This appears as a steep curve to begin, with more and more flattening toward the end. The slope of the washout curve is determined mainly by the rate, tidal volume, FRC, and dead space. The inspired gas distribution index (IDI) offers a more quantitative analysis of the distribution characteristics. (See text.) The test normally lasts 7 minutes, or until the alveolar N_2 concentration has been reduced to less than 1%, or until an expired volume limit has been reached (i.e., 60 L).

tual results of a 7-minute N_2 washout are of little value apart from the tidal volume, dead space, and FRC of the individual patient. Large increases in minute volume can lower $\%N_2$ in the alveoli to near normal levels within the 7-minute limit even though there is marked unevenness of gas distribution.

The graphic method of displaying breath-by-breath washout yields somewhat more diagnostic results. The slope of the curve is determined by the FRC, tidal volume, respiratory dead space, and frequency of breathing. If the N_2 is washed out of the lungs evenly, the curve will appear as a straight line on semilog paper, no matter what the slope (Fig. 4-2). Because the lung is not a perfectly symmetrical organ, the curve is seldom a straight line. The deviation from a straight line is indicative of the extent to which ventilation is uneven.

The data from the washout can be used to derive the index of distribution of inspired gas (IDI) (Fig. 4-3). The IDI is defined as equal to the alveolar ventilation (accumulated over the entire test) divided by the FRC and multiplied by a constant:

$$IDI = \frac{V_{A(tot)}}{FRC\ (k)}$$

where

k = Constant such that an ideal lung (single compartment) will have an IDI equal to 1.00

The technique eliminates the dependence on the tidal volume, rate, and respiratory dead space as determinants of the slope of the washout curve. Total alveolar ventilation can be calculated as follows:

$$V_{A(tot)} = V_{(tot)} - f(V_D)$$

where

$V_{(tot)}$ = Total volume expired during test
V_D = Respiratory dead space
f = Number of breaths

In an ideal lung the IDI equals 1.00, and in normal subjects it is about 1.80 ± 0.2. Obstructive diseases show mean

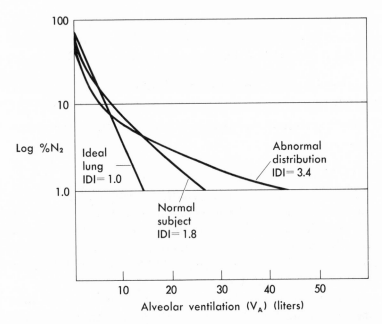

Fig. 4-3. Inspired gas distribution index (IDI). Illustrated is a plot of the logarithm of N_2 concentration versus the alveolar ventilation. The IDI is derived thus:

$$IDI = \frac{V_A}{FRC\ (K)}$$

where

K = Constant equal to the natural log of 72 (see text)

By definition, IDI for an ideal, single-chambered lung is 1.0. Plotting log N_2 concentration against alveolar ventilation instead of total expired volume eliminates dependence on rate, tidal volume, and dead space as determinants of the shape of the washout curve and allows a quantitative measurement of the evenness of distribution. (From Application note AN729, San Diego, Hewlett-Packard Co.)

values of 3.40 ± 0.9. Thus the IDI is a quantitative expression of the gas distribution as analyzed by the multiple-breath nitrogen technique.

Uneven distribution is characteristic of all obstructive disease patterns, with emphysema showing the greatest degree of maldistribution. Pure restrictive patterns often show normal washout values, especially in patients who hyperventilate as a result of restriction. Both the simple multiple-breath N_2 test and the IDI are independent of patient effort.

RADIOXENON (^{133}Xe) (LUNG SCAN)
Description

The radioxenon technique measures the regional distribution of ventilation.

Technique

1. The subject, usually in a sitting position, inhales a normal tidal volume from a reservoir that contains a measured dose of ^{133}Xe (10 to 20 microcuries). The subject then holds his breath for 10 to 20 seconds. During this time photoscintograms are made over the lung fields to determine areas of poor ventilation (Fig. 4-4).

2. The subject may be allowed to rebreathe the gas mixture containing the xenon for a 10- to 15-minute interval, during which serial scintograms are made to determine the rapidity and evenness of equilibration of the radiogas.

3. As a final step, the subject can return to breathing atmospheric gas to cause the ^{133}Xe to be washed out. Serial photoscintograms will indicate those areas that have trapped the xenon during the equilibration phase. Radiation counters placed over various lung zones can be used to determine the relative extent of ventilation (or perfusion) in respective zones by comparisons of the counting rates for each zone.

Significance

Radioxenon is ideal for identifying regional ventilation disorders. It has a half-life of 5.27 days and requires rather sophisticated monitoring equipment, but it is not metabolized by the body and tends to remain in the gas phase. The three types of radioxenon studies just outlined can be done individually or as a series and are helpful diagnostically in cases of pronounced regional differences in ventilation. Regional distribution of inspired gas is dependent on the volume of air in

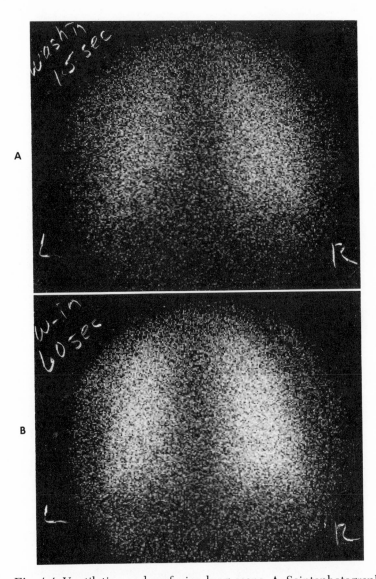

Fig. 4-4. Ventilation and perfusion lung scans. **A,** Scintophotograph showing posteroanterior view of the lung fields after 15 seconds of rebreathing ^{133}Xe. **B,** The same subject after 60 seconds of rebreathing.

Continued.

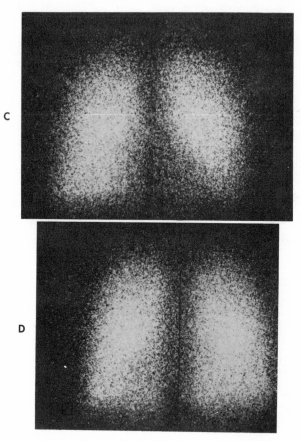

Fig. 4-4, cont'd. C, A normal perfusion lung scan made with micro-aggregated albumin particles treated with 131I (133I MAA), anterior view. **D,** Same subject, posterior view. Ventilation and perfusion lung scans are of maximal diagnostic value when correlated on the same subject. Each offers an index of distribution, and together they provide a measurement of how well blood flow and ventilation match, which is of prime importance in the evaluation of pulmonary disorders. (**A** and **B** courtesy Department of Nuclear Medicine, St. John's Mercy Medical Center, Creve Coeur, Mo.; **C** and **D** from Early, P. J., Razzak, M. A., and Sodee, D. B.: Textbook of nuclear medicine technology, St. Louis, 1969, The C. V. Mosby Co.)

the lungs before the breath and the volume of the breath itself. Differences in regional ventilation can be quantified by calculating the concentration of ^{133}Xe in each lung zone by means of external counters placed over the chest. By comparing radiation counts during an initial breath of ^{133}Xe to counts at the same lung volume after rebreathing, when the concentration of ^{133}Xe is equal in both the lung and the breathing circuit, the fractional concentration of ^{133}Xe during the initial breath can be derived. This fractional concentration can then be stated as a "ventilation index," by expressing it as a percentage of the simultaneous mean concentration of ^{133}Xe in the lungs. The concentration of ^{133}Xe is thus expressed per unit of lung volume, and similar data from different subjects can be compared. Typical values in normal subjects show proportionately greater ventilation in the bases than in the apices. In perfusion lung scans, a similar method can be employed to generate a "perfusion index" for each lung zone. ^{133}Xe studies can be of greatest benefit only if the normal variables, such as body position and tidal volume, are carefully controlled during testing.

SELECTED BIBLIOGRAPHY

Abboud, R., and Morton, J.: Comparison of maximal mid-expiratory flow, flow-volume curves, and nitrogen closing volumes in patients with mild airway obstruction, Am. Rev. Respir. Dis. **111**:405, 1975.

Ball, W. C., Jr., Stewart, P. B., Newsham, L. G., and Bates, D. V.: Regional pulmonary function studies with ^{133}xenon, J. Clin. Invest. **41**:519, 1962.

Bouhuys, A.: Distribution of inspired gas in the lungs. In Fenn, W. O., and Rahn, H., editors: Handbook of physiology—respiration I, Washington, D.C., 1964, American Physiological Society.

Buist, S., and Ross, B.: Predicted values for closing volumes using a modified single-breath nitrogen test, Am. Rev. Respir. Dis. **107**:744, 1973.

Closing volume, Lancet **2**:908, 1972.

Comroe, J. H. and Fowler, W. S.: Lung function studies. VI. Detection of uneven alveolar ventilation during a single breath of oxygen, Am. J. Med. **10**:408, 1951.

Dollfuss, R. E., Milic-Emili, J., and Bates, D. V.: Regional ventilation of the lung studied with boluses of ^{133}xenon, Respir. Physiol. **2**:234, 1967.

Fowler, W. S., Cornish, E. K., and Kety, S. S.: Analysis of alveolar ventilation by pulmonary N_2 clearance curves, J. Clin. Invest. **31**:40, 1952.

McCarthy, D. S., Spencer, R., Greene, R., and Milic-Emili, J.: Measurement of closing volume as a simple and sensitive test for early detection of small airway disease, Am. J. Med. **52**:747, 1972.

Otis, A. B., et. al.: Mechanical factors in distribution of pulmonary ventilation, J. Appl. Physiol. 8:427, 1956.

Report of Informal Session on "Closing Volume" Determinations, Atlantic City, N.J., April, 1972, distributed by the Lung Program, National Heart and Lung Institute.

Secker-Walker, R. H., and Siegal, B. A.: The use of nuclear medicine in the diagnosis of lung disease, Radiol. Clin. North Am. 11:215, 1973.

Shinokazi, T., Abajian, J. C., Jr., Tabakin, B. S., and Hanson, J. S.: Theory of a digital nitrogen washout computer, J. Appl. Physiol. 21:202, 1966.

CHAPTER FIVE

Diffusion tests

CARBON MONOXIDE DIFFUSING CAPACITY (D_{LCO})

Description

Carbon monoxide diffusing capacity measures all the factors that affect the diffusion of a gas across the alveolo-capillary membrane. The D_{LCO} is recorded as milliliters of CO per minute per millimeter of mercury at STPD.

Technique

Carbon monoxide combines with hemoglobin about 210 times more readily than does O_2. In the presence of normal amounts of hemoglobin and normal ventilatory function, the main limiting factor to diffusion is the status of the alveolo-capillary membrane. Small amounts of CO in inspired gas produce measurable changes in the concentration of inspired versus expired gas. There are several methods for determining the D_{LCO} (Table 2). All of the methods measure diffusing capacity according to the equation:

$$D_{LCO} = \frac{\text{ml CO transferred/min}}{\text{Mean } P_{ACO} - \text{Mean capillary } P_{CO}}$$

An additional method of quantifying diffusing capacity simply relates the inspired and expired CO concentrations during normal breathing.

$D_{LCO}SB$ (modified Krogh technique — single breath). The subject inspires a vital capacity breath from a spirometer or reservoir containing a gas mixture of 0.3% CO, 10% He, and the remainder air, and then holds his breath for approximately 10 seconds. The subject then expires, and a sample of alveolar

gas is taken with an end-tidal sampler and analyzed to obtain final fractional CO and He concentrations, $F_{A_{CO_{t2}}}$ and FeHe, respectively (Fig. 5-1). The concentration of CO in alveolar gas at the beginning of the breath hold ($F_{A_{CO_{t1}}}$) is computed by multiplying the initial CO concentration (0.3%) by a factor derived thus:

$$\frac{F_{eHe}}{F_{iHe}}$$

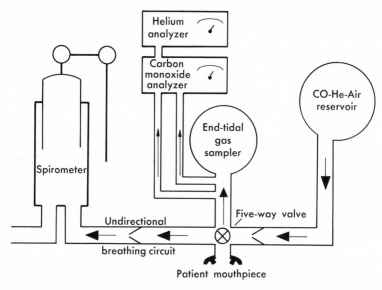

Fig. 5-1. $D_{L_{CO}}$ apparatus. The basic equipment for performing the $D_{L_{CO}}$ test is illustrated. Included is a CO-He-air reservoir, which may be a large volume bag or a demand valve–type system. A five-way valve (which may be automatic) allows rapid switching of breathing gases and directs exhaled gas to the end-tidal sampler or spirometer or both. He and CO analyzers are used to monitor the end-tidal sample, but may be used to determine inspired gas concentrations from the CO-He-air reservoir. Most automated systems include electronic timing circuits, such as that necessary for the $D_{L_{CO}}$ SB breath hold maneuver.

where

F_{eHe} = Exhaled fractional He concentration measured from the end-tidal sample

F_{iHe} = Inspired He concentration (known)

The $D_{LCO}SB$ is then calculated as follows:

$$D_{LCO}SB = \frac{V_A \times 60}{(P_B - 47)(t_2 - t_1)} \times Ln \frac{(F_{ACO_{t1}})}{(F_{ACO_{t2}})}$$

where

V_A = Alveolar volume (STPD)

60 = Correction from seconds to minutes

P_B = Barometric pressure

47 = Water vapor pressure ($P_{H_{20}}$)

$t_2 - t_1$ = Breath hold interval (usually 10 sec)

Ln = Natural logarithm

$F_{ACO_{t1}}$ = fraction of CO in alveolar gas before diffusion (as measured above)

$F_{ACO_{12}}$ = Fraction of CO in alveolar gas at the end of diffusion

Alveolar volume, V_A, must be determined to calculate the volume of CO that diffused, as expressed by the logarithmic ratio. Since the He inspired is simply diluted by the residual volume, V_A can be calculated from the inspired volume and the initial and final He concentrations by a method similar to the closed circuit determination of FRC. Correction must be made for dead space and all lung volumes corrected from ATPS to STPD.

$D_{LCO}SS_1$ *(Filey technique—steady state).* The subject breathes a gas mixture of 0.1% to 0.2% CO in the air for 5 to 6 minutes. During the final 2 minutes, expired gas is collected in a Douglas bag and an arterial blood sample is drawn. The exhaled volume is measured and the expired gas is analyzed for CO, CO_2, and O_2. The arterial blood is analyzed for P_{CO_2}. Steady state diffusing capacity is calculated by the equation:

$$D_{LCO}SS_1 = \frac{\dot{V}_{CO}\ (STPD)}{P_{ACO}}$$

where

$\dot{V}_{CO}$ = ml of CO transferred per minute (STPD)
$P_{A_{CO}}$ = Partial pressure of CO in the alveoli

$\dot{V}_{CO}$ is determined from an analysis of the fractional inspired and expired CO ($F_{I_{CO}}$ and $F_{E_{CO}}$ respectively), the minute volume expired ($\dot{V}_E$), and the inspired and expired N_2 fractions (F_{IN2}, which is known, and F_{EN2}, which is determined indirectly from the fractions of O_2, CO_2, and H_2O vapor in the exhaled gas):

$$\dot{V}_{CO} = \dot{V}_E\left(F_{I_{CO}}\frac{F_{E_{N_2}}}{F_{I_{N_2}}} - F_{E_{CO}}\right)$$

The $P_{A_{CO}}$ is determined using a form of the Bohr equation:

$$P_{A_{CO}} = P_B - 47\left(\frac{F_{E_{CO}} - rF_{I_{CO}}}{1 - r}\right)$$

where

$$r = \frac{P_{a_{CO_2}} - P_{E_{CO_2}}}{P_{a_{CO_2}}}$$

Estimating $P_{A_{CO}}$ in this way avoids the necessity of obtaining a direct alveolar sample.

$D_{L_{CO}}SS_2$ *(end-tidal CO determination).* The $D_{L_{CO}}SS_2$ method is basically the same as the $D_{L_{CO}}SS_1$ in that the volume of CO transferred $\dot{V}_{CO}$ is derived similarly. $P_{A_{CO}}$, however, is determined by taking the average end-tidal CO tension ($P_{ET_{CO}}$) from instantaneous analysis of multiple breaths. The end-tidal value is assumed to be equal to the mean $P_{A_{CO}}$.

$D_{L_{CO}}SS_3$ *(assumed dead space technique).* Again, the $D_{L_{CO}}SS_3$ method resembles the $D_{L_{CO}}SS_1$. $\dot{V}_{CO}$ is determined as in $D_{L_{CO}}SS_1$, but the $P_{A_{CO}}$ is measured differently. The fractional alveolar concentration ($F_{A_{CO}}$), which can be used to derive $P_{A_{CO}}$ when the barometric pressure (P_B) is known, is measured as follows:

$$F_{A_{CO}} = \frac{V_T F_{E_{CO}} - V_D F_{I_{CO}}}{V_T - V_D}$$

where

V_T = Tidal volume
V_D = Dead space volume
$F_{E_{CO}}$ = Fraction of expired CO
$F_{I_{CO}}$ = Fraction of inspired CO

Tidal volume (V_T) is measured by averaging multiple breaths. Dead space (V_D) is often assumed to be equal to 1 ml per pound of body weight. The mechanical dead space of the breathing assembly is subtracted.

$D_{L_{CO}}SS_4$ *(mixed venous P_{CO_2} technique).* $\dot{V}_{CO}$ is obtained as in $D_{L_{CO}}SS_1$. The $P_{A_{CO}}$ is calculated by estimating the mixed venous P_{CO_2} ($P\overline{V}_{CO_2}$) from an equilibration technique and then determining the $P_{A_{CO_2}}$ (alveolar) from the $P\overline{V}_{CO_2}$ and the normal gradient. Once the $P_{A_{CO_2}}$ is derived, an equation similar to that used to determine $P_{A_{CO}}$ in the $D_{L_{CO}}SS_1$ technique can be employed. Using mixed venous P_{CO_2} avoids the necessity of arterial puncture.

$D_{L_{CO}}RB$ *(rebreathing technique).* The subject rebreathes from a reservoir containing a mixture of 0.3% CO, 10% He, and the remainder air for 30 to 60 seconds at a rate of about 30 per minute. After the interval, measurement of the final CO, He, and O_2 concentrations in the reservoir are made. An equation similar to that used for the single-breath technique is used (see p. 67):

$$D_{L_{CO}}RB = \frac{V_S \times 60}{(P_B - 47)(t_2 - t_1)} \times Ln \frac{F_{CO_{t1}}}{F_{CO_{t2}}}$$

where

$\dot{V}_S$ = Volume of the lung reservoir system (initial volume $\times$ $\dfrac{F_{i_{He}}}{F_{e_{He}}}$
60 = Correction for uptake from seconds to minute
P_B = Barometric pressure
47 = Water vapor pressure
$t_1 - t_2$ = Rebreathing interval
$F_{CO_{t1}}$ = Initial CO fraction in reservoir
$F_{CO_{t2}}$ = Final CO fraction reservoir

$D_{LCO}SS_{He}$ *(equilibration−washout method).* The subject rebreathes from a reservoir containing 0.3% CO, 10% He, and the remainder air until equilibrium is reached. Then the subject again breathes room air and the washout of both CO and He are recorded by rapid gas analyzer. During the washout, CO is removed at a rapid rate by diffusion as well as by ventilation, while He is removed more slowly by ventilation alone. The difference in washout rates is caused by the rate of CO diffusion. An equation similar to the $D_{LCO}SB$ equation is used to calculate $D_{LCO}SS_{He}$; a logarithmic expression of the ratio of final He concentration to initial He concentration is included as a factor along with the CO concentration ratio. Analysis of the washout curve normally requires computerization.

Fractional CO uptake (F_{UCO}). The subject inspires a mixture 0.1% CO in air from a reservoir to establish a steady state breathing pattern. He expires into a spirometer or reservoir, from which an average expired CO sample is analyzed. The fractional uptake of CO is expressed as:

$$F_{UCO} = \frac{F_{ICO} - F_{ECO}}{F_{ICO}}$$

where

F_{ICO} = Fraction of inspired CO
F_{ECO} = Fraction of expired CO

The resultant fraction may be multiplied by 100 and expressed as a percentage. The level of minute ventilation, $\dot{V}_E$, is critical to valid determination of F_{UCO} and should be monitored closely.

Membrane diffusion coefficient (D_m) and capillary blood volume (V_c). The subject performs two $D_{LCO}SB$ tests, each at a different level of alveolar P_{O_2}. The first $D_{LCO}SB$ is performed as outlined on p. 65. The subject then breathes a high concentration of oxygen (balance N_2) for approximately 5 minutes. He then immediately exhales to RV and performs the second $D_{LCO}SB$ maneuver. The D_{LCO} values are calculated for both the air and oxygen breathing maneuvers. The total resistance to D_{LCO} at two different alveolar P_{O_2}s is then used to calculate the resistance caused by the alveolocapillary membrane (D_m) and the resistance caused by the rate of chemical combination with hemoglobin (Hb) and transfer into the red blood cell (θV_c) according to the equation:

$$1/D_{LCO} = 1/D_m + 1/\theta V_c$$

where

$1/D_{LCO}$ = Reciprocal of diffusing capacity, or resistance
$1/D_m$ = Alveolocapillary membrane resistance
$1/\theta V_c$ = Resistance caused by the red blood cell membrane and rate of reaction with Hb
θ = Transfer rate of CO per ml of capillary blood
V_c = Capillary blood volume

Because CO and O_2 compete for binding sites on Hb, measurement of diffusion of CO at different levels of P_{O_2} can be used to distinguish resistance caused by the alveolor capillary membrane from resistance caused by the red blood cell membrane and Hb reaction rate. V_c is presumed to remain the same for both tests, but θ varies in response to changes in P_{O_2}. By plotting θ at two points against $1/D_{LCO}$ and extrapolating back to zero (as if no O_2 were present) the resistance caused by the alveolocapillary membrane can be calculated.

Significance

The average value for resting subjects by the single-breath method is 25 ml CO/min/mm Hg (STPD). Values derived by one of the steady state methods are usually slightly less in normal subjects. Females show slightly lower normal values, presumably in correlation with smaller normal lung volumes. D_{LCO} values can increase 2 to 3 times in normal individuals during exercise.

Table 2 compares the advantages and disadvantages of the testing methods discussed in this chapter.

In general, the $D_{LCO}SB$ is the most widely used method because of its simplicity and noninvasive nature. However,

Table 2. Advantages and disadvantages of testing methods

Method	Technique	Advantages	Disadvantages	Application
$D_{L_{CO}}SB$ (breath-hold)	He and CO analysis relatively simple; 10-second breath-hold	Easy calculations; simple; fast; no CO-Hb back pressure; can be automated	Sensitive to distribution of ventilation and $\dot{V}/\dot{Q}$; "non-physiologic"; not practical for exercise	Screening and clinical application; good standardization
$D_{L_{CO}}SS_1$ (Filey technique)	CO, CO_2, O_2 analysis; arterial blood sample; relatively simple	Most accurate steady state method; good for exercise testing	Arterial puncture and blood gas analysis; sensitive to uneven $\dot{V}/\dot{Q}$	Clinical application; exercise testing
$D_{L_{CO}}SS_2$ (end-tidal CO)	End-tidal sample, $F_{U_{CO}}$ simultaneously; CO analysis only	No arterial puncture or breath hold; easy calculation	CO-Hb back pressure; V_t must be maintained high; very sensitive to $\dot{V}/\dot{Q}$; sensitive to CO-Hb	Fast, easy screening and clinical method; not used for exercise studies
$D_{L_{CO}}SS_3$ (assumed V_D)	CO analysis (slow or fast); large V_T improves accuracy	Relatively simple calculations; good for exercise study	Large error if V_T is too small; sensitive to CO-Hb	Screening and clinical applications; exercise studies

$D_{LCO}SS_4$ (mixed venous P_{CO_2})	CO, CO_2 analysis; rebreathing required	No arterial puncture; easy calculations; slow CO analyzer acceptable	Sensitive to CO-Hb, rebreathing must be closely controlled	Not yet widely used clinically
D_{LCO} RB (rebreathing)	He and CO analysis (rapid); rebreathing required	Less sensitive to V_A than $D_{LCO}SB$; less sensitive to $\dot{V}/\dot{Q}$ abnormalities	Complex calculations; rapid CO and He analyzers required; sensitive to CO-Hb	Clinically applicable; provides most accurate D_{LCO}
$D_{LCO}SSHe$ (equilibration washout)	CO, He analysis rapid; sequencing required	Eliminates V_A, $\dot{V}/\dot{Q}$, and distribution problems	Complex calculations (computerized)	Research applications
F_{UCO} (fractional CO uptake)	CO analysis; may be done with $D_{LCO}SS_2$	Simple; CO analysis of inspired and expired gas only	Sensitive to minute volume, $\dot{V}/\dot{Q}$, and V_D/V_T	Screening or correlation to $D_{LCO}SS_2$
$1/D_m + 1/\theta V_c$ (membrane and red blood cell resistance)	$D_{LCO}SB$ repeated before and after O_2 breathing	Differentiates membrane from red blood cell components; calculates capillary volume, V_c	Complex calculations; estimates of alveolar P_{O_2} critical	Research with limited clinical applications

because breath holding is not a physiologic maneuver and the measured value of D_{LCO} varies with lung volume while holding the breath, the $D_{LCO}SB$ may not be an accurate description of diffusing capacity.

The steady state methods, $D_{LCO}SS_{1-4}$, all use various methods of estimating the mean alveolar P_{CO}. $D_{LCO}SS_1$ probably has the broadest application of the steady state methods. The widespread availability of arterial blood gas analysis has enabled more common usage. The end-tidal CO ($D_{LCO}SS_2$) is gaining in popularity because of the availability of fast response CO analyzers (see Chapter 8) and is often done in combination with the fractional uptake of CO (F_{UCO}). The $D_{LCO}SS_3$ (assumed dead space) is commonly used for measurement of diffusion capacity during exercise, since small differences in the assumed V_D become less significant when the tidal volume increases. All of the steady state methods can be applied to exercise testing.

The rebreathing method is more complicated in terms of the calculations involved but offers the advantage of a normal breathing pattern without arterial puncture. $D_{LCO}RB$ is less sensitive to $\dot{V}/\dot{Q}$ abnormalities and uneven ventilation distribution than either the $D_{LCO}SB$ or the steady state methods. The rebreathing method and the steady state methods may suffer some inaccuracy because of a build-up of CO-Hb in the capillary blood and the resultant "back pressure." Capillary P_{CO} is routinely assumed to be zero, but the actual alveolo-capillary gradient at the time of testing can be estimated, though with some difficulty.

The equilibration-washout method, $D_{LCO}SSHe$, is the most sophisticated technique. It is relatively insensitive to $\dot{V}/\dot{Q}$ and ventilation abnormalities but requires computerization and is probably limited to research applications.

Calculation of the membrane and red blood cell components of diffusion resistance has revealed that each component accounts for approximately half of the total resistance.

The D_{LO2} may be estimated from the D_{LCO} by multiplying the $D_{LCO} \times 1.23$, although the D_{LCO} is normally reported clinically.

Since D_{LCO} is directly related to alveolar volume, expression of this relationship is often useful in differentiating disease processes in which there may be decreased D_{LCO} as a result of loss of lung volume (restrictive) from those in which decreased D_{LCO} is caused by uneven $\dot{V}/\dot{Q}$ or uneven distribution of inspired gas to alveolar volume (obstructive). As an index, the measured D_{LCO} may be divided by the lung volume at which the measurement was made to obtain an expression of diffusing capacity per unit of lung volume. This is recorded as the D_L/V_L or D_L/V_A and may be accomplished easily since alveolar volume must be calculated to derive the D_{LCO}.

Some of the other factors that can influence the D_{LCO} are:
1. Hematocrit and hemoglobin (decreased Hct and Hb decrease the D_{LCO})
2. Alveolar P_{CO_2} (increased P_{CO_2} raises D_{LCO})
3. Body position (supine position increases D_{LCO})
4. Pulmonary capillary blood volume (V_c)

In general, diffusing capacity is decreased in alveolar fibrosis associated with sarcoidosis, asbestosis, berylliosis, oxygen toxicity, or edema. These states are usually categorized as "diffusion defects," although they are probably more closely related to loss of lung volume or capillary bed. D_{LCO} is decreased in emphysema because of the decrease in surface area, loss of capillary bed, increased distance from the terminal bonchiole to the alveolocapillary membrane, and mismatching of ventilation and blood flow. Diffusion capacity is decreased by space-occupying lesions and lung resection.

SELECTED BIBLIOGRAPHY

Bates, D. V., Macklem, P. T., and Christie, R. V.: Respiratory function in disease, Philadelphia, 1971, W. B. Saunders Co.

Burrows, B., Kasih, J. E., Niden, A. H., and Narclay, W. R.: Clinical usefulness of the single breath pulmonary diffusing capacity test, Am. Rev. Respir. Dis. **84**:789, 1961.

Filey, G. F., MacIntosh, D. J., and Wright, G. W.: Carbon monoxide uptake and pulmonary diffusing capacity in normal subjects at rest and during exercise, J. Clin. Invest. **33**:530, 1954.

Forster, R. E.: Exchange of gases between alveolar air and pulmonary capillary blood; pulmonary diffusing capacity, Physiol. Rev. **37**:391, 1957.

Forster, R. E.: Diffusion of gases. In Fenn, W. O., and Rahn, H., editors:

Handbook of physiology—respiration I, Washington, D.C., 1964, American Physiological Society.

Marks, A., et al.: Clinical determination of the diffusion capacity of the lungs: comparison of methods in normal subjects and patients with "alveolar-capillary block" syndrome, Am. J. Med. **22:**51, 1957.

McNeill, R. S., Rankin, J., and Forster, R. E.: The diffusing capacity of the pulmonary membrane and the pulmonary capillary blood volume in cardiopulmonary disease, Clin. Sci. **17:**465, 1958.

Ogilvie, C. M., et al.: A standardized breath holding technique for the clinical measurement of the diffusing capacity of the lung for carbon monoxide, J. Clin. Invest. **36:**1, 1957.

Rankin, J.: Evaluation of alveolar-capillary diffusion. In Clinical cardiopulmonary physiology, New York, 1960, Grune & Stratton, Inc.

West, J. B.: Pulmonary pathophysiology: the essentials, Baltimore, 1977, The Williams & Wilkins, Co.

West, J. B.: Respiratory physiology: the essentials, Baltimore 1974, The Williams & Wilkins Co.

CHAPTER SIX

Ventilation/blood flow tests

BLOOD GAS ANALYSIS
ARTERIAL OXYGEN TENSION (P_{aO_2})
Description

The P_{aO_2} is a measurement of the partial pressure exerted by O_2 in arterial blood. It is recorded in millimeters of mercury.

Technique

The arterial oxygen tension is measured by submitting whole arterial blood, obtained by anaerobic arterial puncture, to a membrane-covered platinum electrode, which reacts with O_2 molecules. (See Fig. 8-13.) The blood is collected in a heparinized syringe and sealed from the atmosphere immediately. The sample should be stored on ice if analysis is not to be done within 15 or 20 minutes.

Significance

The P_{aO_2} of a healthy young adult varies from 85 to 100 mm Hg. The P_{aO_2} can be increased with normal lungs by hyperventilation, to values as high as 120 mm Hg. Normal subjects breathing 100% O_2 exhibit a P_{aO_2} in excess of 600 mm Hg. Decreased P_{aO_2} can result from (1) hypoventilation, (2) diffusion defects, and (3) ventilation/blood flow imbalances.

The severity of impairment of arterial oxygenation is indicated by the P_{aO_2} at rest. Severe obstructive or restrictive diseases will show a decreased oxygen tension in resting subjects, occasionally as low as 40 mm Hg. Less advanced pulmonary disease may show little decrease in P_{aO_2} if hyperventilation is present. However, analysis of P_{aO_2} during exercise often displays a decrease in arterial oxygen tension commensurate with the extent of the disease process. The P_{aO_2} may be decreased for nonpulmonary reasons such as (1) inadequate atmospheric O_2, (2) anatomic shunts (intracardiac), or (3) neuromuscular hypoventilation. The P_{aO_2} is of greatest value when correlated with adequate ventilation ($\dot{V}_E$, V_T, V_D) and lung volume tests (VC, RV, TLC). The main disadvantage is the necessity of arterial puncture.

ARTERIAL OXYGEN SATURATION (S_{aO_2})
Description

Arterial oxygen saturation measures the amount of oxygen in milliliters combined with hemoglobin as related to the maximum capacity of that same hemoglobin for binding O_2. This ratio of content to capacity is expressed as a percentage.

Technique

Oxygen saturation of hemoglobin can be measured in three ways. (1) The O_2 content of arterial blood is measured, and the blood is exposed to the atmosphere so that the Hb may combine with atmospheric O_2, after which the content is measured again. Saturation is determined after corrections for dissolved O_2 are made. (2) The O_2 saturation can also be measured spectrophotometrically by analyzing the ratio of oxyhemoglobin to total hemoglobin. (3) Saturation can also be obtained by ear oximetry.

Significance

The percent of saturation for a healthy young adult with a P_{aO_2} of 95 mm Hg is approximately 97%. Because of the shape of the oxygen-hemoglobin dissociation curve, large changes in P_{aO_2} effect small changes in saturation, above partial pressures of 70 mm Hg. Therefore the P_{aO_2} is a more sensitive indicator of ventilation in lungs without gross abnormalities. As the partial pressure of O_2 falls below 50 mm Hg, the degree to which Hb binds O_2 decreases rapidly. In essence, the percent of saturation is a measure of the relationship between O_2 and Hb.

The percent of saturation of mixed venous blood is 75% (P_vO_2 = 40 mm Hg). As arterial saturation falls from 97% toward 75%, the failure of the lungs to oxygenate mixed venous blood is indicated. The percent of saturation does not indicate the O_2 content of arterial blood, which is determined by the concentration of Hb as well as the P_{aO_2}.

ARTERIAL CO_2 TENSION (P_{aCO_2})
Description

The P_{aCO_2} is a measure of the partial pressure exerted by CO_2 in arterial blood. The measurement is expressed in mm Hg.

Technique

The P_{aCO_2} is measured by submitting arterial blood to a glass electrode covered with a membrane in which the CO_2 combines with water to form H_2CO_3 (carbonic acid). The dissociation of H_2CO_3 into H^+ and HCO_3^- is measured by electrode and is proportional to the P_{aCO_2}. (See Fig. 8-13.) Again the arterial blood must be kept in an anaerobic state until analysis.

Significance

The P_{aCO_2} of a healthy young adult is approximately 40 mm Hg (35 to 45 mm Hg). The P_{aCO_2} is an index of alveolar ventilation. A rise in P_{aCO_2} is usually associated with hypoventilation, a fall with hyperventilation. Because CO_2 diffuses twenty times as readily as O_2, small changes in the ventilatory pattern or distribution of gas will show little or no change in P_{aCO_2}. Patients with localized lesions often hyperventilate functional alveoli and maintain a normal CO_2 tension. An increase in P_{aCO_2} means that at least a major portion of the lung is hypoventilated. Diffusion defects rarely raise the P_{aCO_2}. The carbon dioxide tension may be normal or low even in moderately advanced pulmonary disease. The P_{aCO_2} is most valuable as a diagnostic tool when correlated to the minute ventilation, tidal volume, rate, P_{ao_2}, and pH. The minute volume necessary to maintain a given P_{aco_2} is indicative of the amount of functional lung tissue. For example, a normal CO_2 tension accompanied by a large minute ventilation (15 to 20 liters) points to a large amount of wasted ventilation or dead space. The correlation of oxygen and carbon dioxide tensions often gives a key to the nature of ventilatory impairments. Subjects with high P_{aco_2}s and low P_{ao_2}s have the most severe derangements because a sufficiently large part of the pulmonary tissue is involved, so that even the fast-diffusing CO_2 cannot be eliminated efficiently. This is common in advanced emphysema, chronic bronchitis, and acute asthmatic episodes. A gas exchange system that cannot remove CO_2 can very rarely arterialize mixed venous blood, even in the presence of increased inspired oxygen concentrations. Similarly, a low P_{aco_2} along with a low P_{ao_2} indicates that although enough mixed venous blood is passing through the pulmonary capillaries to cause an oxygenation defect, a sufficiently large portion of the gas exchange mechanism is working to remove an adequate amount of CO_2. In effect, hyperventilation caused by hypoxemia can often cause inappropriate removal of CO_2. The relation of the P_{aco_2} to pH and HCO_3^- defines the acid-base status of the body (Table 3).

The only disadvantage of measuring P_{aco_2} is the required arterial blood sample. End-tidal P_{CO_2} is sometimes used to estimate P_{aco_2}.

ARTERIAL pH
Description

pH is the negative logarithm of the hydrogen ion (H^+) concentration used as a positive number. pH is recorded in pH units ranging from 1 to 14, 1 being most acid, 14 being most basic, and 7 being the pH of water, or neutral.

Technique

Arterial pH is measured by submitting arterial blood to a glass electrode under anaerobic conditions. (See Fig. 8-13.)

Table 3. Acid-base status

Status	pH	P_{CO_2}	HCO_3^-
Simple disorders			
Metabolic acidosis	Low	Normal	Low
Metabolic alkalosis	High	Normal	High
Respiratory acidosis	Low	High	Normal
Respiratory alkalosis	High	Low	Normal
Compensated disorders			
Compensated respiratory acidosis, or metabolic alkalosis	Normal*	High	High
Compensated metabolic acidosis, or respiratory alkalosis	Normal*	Low	Low
Combined disorders			
Metabolic/respiratory acidosis	Low	High	Low
Metabolic/respiratory alkalosis	High	Low	High

*Compensation cannot return values to within normal limits in severe acid-base disturbances.

Correction must be made for temperature changes. The pH can also be determined indirectly if the plasma HCO_3^- and P_{aCO_2} are known, by application of the Henderson-Hasselbalch equation:

$$pH = pK + \log \frac{(HCO_3^-)}{(CO_2)}$$

where

pK = Negative log of dissociation constant for carbonic acid (6.1)
(HCO_3^-) = Molar concentration of serum bicarbonate
(CO_2) = Molar concentration of CO_2

To simplify actual calculation, the P_{aCO_2}, which can be measured directly, is substituted for (CO_2), and the total $CO_2 - P_{aCO_2}$ (0.03) is substituted for (HCO_3^-); 0.03 is a solubility factor introduced to simplify handling the P_{aCO_2}. The equation then becomes:

$$pH = pK + \log \frac{(\text{Total CO}_2 - 0.03[P_{aCO_2}])}{0.03(P_{aCO_2})}$$

Significance

The pH of arterial blood of a healthy young adult ranges from 7.35 to 7.45. As the pH falls below 7.35, the blood becomes more acidic; as it rises above 7.45, the blood becomes increasingly alkaline, or basic.

Since one of the main functions of the lungs is to remove CO_2, their ability to function is directly related to the acid-base status of the body. When CO_2 is retained, pH falls, and the resulting acidosis is respiratory in origin. Likewise, if CO_2 is "blown off," respiratory alkalosis ensues (Table 3). Diagnostically, arterial pH is of greatest value when correlated to minute volume and P_{aCO_2}. Increased P_{aCO_2} normally causes acidosis, except in the presence of renal compensation (retention and production of bicarbonate). If the acidosis is of metabolic origin (diabetes, etc.), hyperventilation and a fall in P_{aCO_2} normally occur. Chronic obstructive pulmonary disease and chronic CO_2 retention often result in grossly exaggerated blood gas values and HCO_3^- levels with a resultant pH close to normal limits because of chronic compensation. Acute ventilatory impairment (pneumonia, etc.) often shows little or no renal compensation; when present, it is seldom as pronounced as in long-term compensation. Hence lung function and P_{aCO_2} in particular often serve to define acid-base disorders.

Arterial blood is normally used for pH determinations because venous blood is slightly more acidic.

SINGLE-BREATH CO₂ ELIMINATION
Description

The single-breath CO_2 test measures the uniformity of both ventilation and pulmonary blood flow. It is recorded as a percentage.

Technique

The subject exhales into a CO_2 analyzer that continuously monitors the concentration of CO_2 in expired gas. The change in CO_2 concentration is recorded graphically, as is done in the single-breath nitrogen elimination test (Fig. 6-1). The percentage change over a given interval after the dead space gas has been exhaled is measured to index the uniformity of ventilation to blood flow.

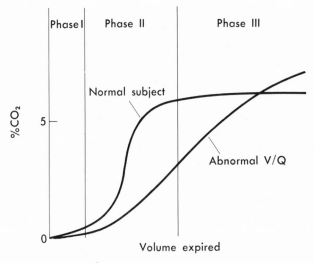

Fig. 6-1. Carbon dioxide elimination. A plot of expired CO_2 concentration against expired volume yields a curve distinctly similar to a single-breath nitrogen elimination curve. Three phases can be defined: *Phase I* includes the expiration of dead space gas containing little CO_2; *Phase II* shows an abrupt rise in %CO_2 as mixed bronchial and alveolar air is expired; *Phase III* shows the typical plateau as alveolar gas is monitored. Also illustrated is an elimination curve typical of abnormal ventilation/blood flow ratios. When different parts of the lung have different CO_2 concentrations, and different parts empty at different rates, the carbon dioxide elimination curve will show a constant rise during the entire expiration. The single-breath N_2 test indicates abnormality of ventilation; the CO_2 elimination test indicates abnormal blood flow *as well as* abnormal ventilation. If ventilation shifts to match uneven blood flow (or vice versa), the elimination curve will assume a more normal S shape.

Significance

In normal individuals the concentration of CO_2 in expired gas rises to a plateau as alveolar gas is expired and remains more or less constant. The single-breath CO_2 test will show a continuous rise with expired volume in lungs that exhibit uneven ventilation and at the same time determine if the blood flow matches the distribution of ventilation. If all parts of the lungs emptied CO_2 at exactly the same rate, there would be no rise in the concentration of carbon dioxide. But since lungs with ventilation and blood flow imbalances empty CO_2 at varying rates, the CO_2 concentration rises as more and more of the vital capacity is expired. The slope of the CO_2 elimination curve (Fig. 6-1) is determined by the extent of variation in ventilation as compared with perfusion. The absolute concentrations of CO_2 expired depend on various factors, but the quantitative value of the test is not influenced by the magnitude of the CO_2 concentration, only the amount of change.

The single-breath CO_2 test is difficult insofar as it requires a CO_2 analyzer and a recording device for plotting CO_2 concentration against expired volume. Since it is not a strictly quantitative analysis, it is often replaced by a calculation of the physiologic dead space (Chapter 2), or the percent shunt. With appropriate facilities, the radioxenon test and perfusion lung scan can be used to obtain similar qualitative judgments of ventilation/blood flow inequalities.

CLINICAL SHUNT CALCULATION $(\dot{Q}_s/\dot{Q}_t)$
Description

The clinical shunt calculation is a measurement of the fraction of blood that traverses the pulmonary system without participating in gas exchange. It is recorded as a percent of the total capillary blood flow.

Technique

The subject is allowed to breathe 100% O_2 for at least 20 minutes at atmospheric pressure so that all N_2 is washed out of the lungs and the hemoglobin can become completely saturated. The percent shunt can then be calculated thus:

$$\frac{\dot{Q}_s}{\dot{Q}_t} \times 100 = \frac{(P_{A_{O_2}} - P_{a_{O_2}}) \times 0.0031}{C(a\text{-}v)O_2 + (P_{A_{O_2}} - P_{a_{O_2}}) \times 0.0031}$$

where

$\dot{Q}_s/\dot{Q}_t$ = Ratio of shunted blood to total perfusion
$P_{A_{O_2}}$ = Alveolar O_2 tension
$P_{a_{O_2}}$ = Arterial O_2 tension
$C(a\text{-}v)O_2$ = Arteriovenous oxygen content difference
0.0031 = Conversion factor to vol% for O_2

Alveolar oxygen tension, breathing 100% O_2, can be estimated as follows:

$$P_{A_{O_2}} = P_B - P_{A_{H_2O}} - 0.8\ P_{A_{CO_2}}$$

where

P_B = Barometric pressure
$P_{A_{H_2O}}$ = Partial pressure of water vapor at body temperature (47 mm Hg)
$P_{A_{CO_2}}$ = Alveolar CO_2 tension (estimated from arterial P_{CO_2})
0.8 = Correction based on respiratory exchange ratio

The shunt equation is accurate only when the hemoglobin is completely saturated, and this requires a $P_{a_{O_2}}$ of greater than 150 mm Hg. This is usually easily accomplished by breathing pure O_2. (See the Appendix for a more detailed description of the technique.)

Significance

Normally, less than 5% of the cardiac output is shunted. The accuracy of the shunt measurement just outlined depends on the accuracy of the P_{O_2} determinations, since in small shunts the Hb still becomes 100% saturated, and the difference in P_{O_2} is a result of the amount of O_2 dissolved. The actual value for percent of shunt depends largely on the value of the oxygen content difference between arterial and mixed venous blood ($C[a\text{-}v]O_2$) used in the denominator of the equation. Since the a-v content difference is determined not only by the status of the pulmonary system, but by the cardiac output and perfusion status, the value used in the equation should ideally be measured rather than estimated. Arterial content can be measured easily from a sample taken from a peripheral artery, but mixed venous content can only be measured accurately from a sample taken from the pulmonary artery. In subjects in whom the right heart has not been catheterized, an estimated value must be used. Values of 4.5 to 5.0 vols% are reasonable a-v differences in patients with good cardiac outputs and perfusion states. Values of 3.5 vols% are probably more realistic differences in patients who are critically ill.

In instances when the a-v content difference cannot be reliably estimated or when the Hb cannot be maximally saturated by breathing 100% oxygen, the alveolar-arterial oxygen gradient, $A\text{-}aDO_2$, may be used as an index of the matching of ventilation to blood flow. The calculation of percent shunt does not derive any absolute values for Q_s, but if the cardiac output ($\dot{Q}$) is known, $\dot{Q}_s$ can be determined simply. Increased shunting (percent) is indicative of low ventilation in relation to blood flow, as is often found in both obstructive and restrictive disease patterns. It should be noted, however, that even in advanced obstructive or severe restrictive diseases, blood flow may be decreased to the areas of poor ventilation by the lesions themselves or by compensatory mechanisms. In these cases there will be a minimal amount of shunting, even though severe ventilatory impairment may exist. Perhaps most common is increased shunting caused by acute disease patterns such as atelectasis or aspiration of particulate matter or pulmonary hemangiomas in the presence of neoplasms.

The shunt measurement's main disadvantage is that inhalation of pure O_2 for 20 minutes is often contraindicated in patients whose main respiratory drive is hypoxemia. In addition, breathing pure O_2 washes N_2 out of the lungs completely. In subjects in whom certain lung units may be poorly ventilated, the washout of N_2 plus the removal of O_2 by perfusing blood flow may reduce the size of alveoli to their critical limit and cause alveolar collapse. The net effect of the "nitrogen shunting" may be clinical shunt values that are falsely high, since a certain amount of shunting was induced by the testing procedure.

Measurement of the clinical shunt is often correlated with determination of the dead space to tidal volume ratio. (See Chapter 2.)

RADIOXENON ELIMINATION (^{133}Xe)
Description

Radioxenon elimination evaluates the uniformity of ventilation to blood flow by visual assessment of the removal of dissolved ^{133}Xe by the lungs.

Technique

^{133}Xe dissolved in normal saline is injected intravenously, dosage being about 5 to 10 microcuries. As the blood carrying the dissolved xenon enters the pulmonary capillaries, the gas begins to diffuse out because of the relatively small amounts of xenon present in alveolar gas. More than 95% of the gas comes out of solution and enters the alveoli in the gas phase. Photoscintograms must be taken with the subject holding his breath.

Significance

Radioxenon elimination offers a qualitative assessment of regional ventilation/blood flow dynamics. Only ventilated *and* perfused alveoli will show up during the breath holding, a true indicator of which regions are ventilated as well as perfused.

The disadvantages of this type of scan are that dissolved ^{133}Xe is relatively difficult to handle, since it comes out of solution so easily, and only one view can be obtained because of the breath holding. Many clinicians prefer combined perfusion lung scans and ventilation lung scans, so that the four normal views can be obtained.

SELECTED BIBLIOGRAPHY

Anthionisen, N. R., Dolowick, M. B., and Bates, D. V.: Steady state measurement of regional ventilation to perfusion ratios in normal man, J. Clin. Invest. **45:**1349, 1966.

Comroe, J. H.: Physiology of respiration, Chicago, 1965, Year Book Medical Publishers, Inc.

Comroe, J. H., Jr., Forster, R. E., Dubois, A. B., Briscoe, W. A., and Carlsen, E.: The lung: clinical physiology and pulmonary function tests, Chicago, 1962, Year Book Medical Publishers, Inc.

Harrison, R. A., Davison, R., Shapiro, B. A., and Mayers, S. N.: Reassessment of the assumed a-v oxygen content difference in the shunt calculation, Anesth. Analg. **54:**198, 1975.

Marks, A., Chervony, I., Lankford, R., et al.: Ventilation-perfusion relationship in humans measured by scintillation scanning, J. Nucl. Med. **9:**450, 1968.

Rahn, H., and Farhi, L. E.: Ventilation, perfusion, and gas exchange—the V_A/Q concept. In Fenn, W. O., and Rahn, H., editors: Handbook of physiology—respiration I, Washington, D.C., 1964, American Physiological Society.

Severinghaus, J. W., and Bradley, A. F.: Electrodes for blood P_{O_2} and P_{CO_2} determinations, J. Appl. Physiol. **13:**515, 1958.

Severinghaus, J. W., an dStupfel, M.: Alveolar deadspace as an index of distribution of blood flow in pulmonary capillaries, J. Appl. Physiol. **10:**335, 1957.

Shapiro, B. A.: Clinical application of blood gases, ed. 2, Chicago, 1977, Year Book Medical Publishers, Inc.

West, J. B.: Distribution of gas and blood in the normal lungs, Br. Med. Bull. **19:**53, 1963.

West, J. B., et al.: Measurement of the ventilation-perfusion ratio inequality in the lung by the analysis of a single expirate, Clin. sci. **16:**529, 1957.

West, J. B.: Pulmonary pathophysiology: the essentials, Baltimore, 1977, The Williams & Wilkins Co.

West, J. B.: Respiratory physiology: the essentials, Baltimore, 1974, The Williams & Wilkins Co.

CHAPTER SEVEN

Testing regimens

The majority of pulmonary function tests measure functional relationships of various parts of the pulmonary anatomy. The diagnosis of pulmonary disorders requires careful evaluation of even more carefully constructed testing regimens. Too often, accurate diagnoses are lacking because of inappropriate testing or insufficient pulmonary history. Appropriate guidelines reduce the confusion that can result from poorly constructed testing regimens.

PULMONARY HISTORY

Basic to accurate diagnosis on any level — physician's office, general hospital laboratory, or cardiopulmonary laboratory — is a background of information pertinent to possible pulmonary disorders. An ordered array of questions that can be easily answered by the subject is the most useful type of history. Following are examples of a questionnaire-type pulmonary history:

1. Age _____   Sex   ☐ M   ☐ F   Height _____   Weight _____
2. **Family History**
   Tuberculosis _____
   COPD _____
   Asthma   _____
   Cancer   _____
   Other   _____
3. **Personal and family history**
   Tuberculosis _____
   COPD _____
   Asthma   _____

Recurrent infections _____

Colds _____

Pneumonia _____

Allergies _____

4. **Personal situation**

Occupation _____

Smoking habits _____

Residence _____

Other contributory factors _____

5. **Present illness/chief complaint**

Dyspnea _____

Dyspnea on exertion _____

Dyspnea related to body position _____

Cough (productive/nonproductive) _____

Hemoptysis _____

6. **Subject disposition at time of test**

Dyspneic _____

Coughing _____

Cyanotic _____

Apprehensive _____

Cooperative/uncooperative _____

7. **General comments** _____

_____

_____

_____

_____

An outline history of this type provides an intelligence base for evaluation of the various tests. In instances in which the physician performs the test, such a history may be redundant if a medical history is available. However, in many instances, pulmonary function testing is performed by ancillary personnel, and then the pulmonary history becomes an essential part of the testing regimen.

CLINIC OR PHYSICIAN'S OFFICE REGIMEN

Following are desirable if not essential tests for basic preliminary or screening purposes:

Lung volumes	*Pulmonary mechanics*
Vital capacity	FVC
Ventilation	FEV_T
Tidal volume (V_T)	FEV_T
Respiratory rate (f)	$FEF_{25\%-75\%}$ or $FEF_{200-1200}$
Minute volume ($\dot{V}_E$)	MVV

GENERAL HOSPITAL LABORATORY

Lung volumes	*Pulmonary mechanics*
Vital capacity	FVC
Inspiratory capacity	FEV
Expiratory reserve	FEV_T
volume	$FEV_{T\%}$
Functional residual volume	$FEF_{25\%-75\%}$ or $FEF_{200-1200}$
(FRC)	Peak flow (PEFR)
Residual volume (RV)	MVV
Total lung capacity	Flow-volume curves
(TLC)	*Gas distribution*
RV/TLC ratio	Single-breath N_2
Ventilation	7-minute N_2 washout
Tidal volume (V_T)	*Diffusion*
Respiratory rate (f)	D_{LCO} single-breath or steady
Minute volume $\dot{V}_E$	(state)
Respiratory dead space	*Ventilation/blood flow*
(V_D)	Arterial blood gases
Alveolar ventilation (V_A)	Percent shunt
	V_D/V_T ratio

CARDIOPULMONARY LABORATORY

Lung volumes
  Vital capacity
  Inspiratory capacity
  Expiratory reserve volume
  Functional residual volume (FRC)
  Residual volume (RV)
  Total lung capacity (TLC)
  RV/TLC ratio
  Thoracic gas volume (TGV)

Ventilation
    Tidal volume (V_T)
    Respiratory rate (f)
    Minute volume ($\dot{V}_E$)
    Respiratory dead space (V_D)
    Alveolar ventilation (V_A)
    CO_2 and O_2 response
Pulmonary mechanics
    FVC
    FEV_T
    $FEV_{T\%}$
    $FEF_{25\%-75\%}$ or $FEF_{200-1200}$
    Peak flow (PEFR)
    MVV
    Compliance (C_L) and frequency dependence (FDC)
    Airway resistance (R_{aw}) and conductance (G_{aw})
    Flow-volume curves (MEFV)
    Volume of isoflow (Viso$\dot{V}$)
Gas distribution
    Single-breath N_2 (SBN_2) and closing volume (CV) or
        closing capacity (CC)
    7-minute N_2 washout and IDI
    Radioxenon distribution and perfusion lung scans
Diffusion
    $D_{L_{CO}}$ (single-breath or steady state)
    $1/D_m$ and $1/\theta V_c$
Ventilation/blood flow
    Arterial blood gases
    Clinical shunt
    Radioxenon clearance (^{133}Xe)
    Exercise testing

To standardize procedures and to ensure the greatest accuracy, recording of test results should follow a format as outlined in Fig. 7-1. Test results are reported in conjunction with the appropriate predicted normals and a corresponding percent of normal. Many studies providing predicted normal values are available for the more common pulmonary function

Test	Subject	Predicted	% Normal
Lung Volumes			
VC i-e			
e-i			
FRC			
RV			
TLC			
RV/TLC x 100%			
Ventilation			
Vt			
$\dot{V}_E$			
f			
Pulmonary Mechanics			
FVC			
FEV 0.5			
FEV 1.0			
FEV 1.0%			
FEF 25-75%			
MVV			
Arterial Blood Gases			
PaO_2			
% Sat.			
$PaCO_2$			
pH			
Distribution			
Single Breath N_2			
7 Minute N_2			
Miscellaneous			

PATIENT_____ SEX _____

AGE _____ HEIGHT _____ WEIGHT _____

INTERPRETATION:

DIAGNOSIS:

Interpreted by_____

Performed by_____

Fig. 7-1. Typical data record sheet.

tests. The standard deviation or standard error of estimate (SEE) for any predicted normal should be taken into consideration in the final evaluation of the extent of lung dysfunction (Fig. 7-1).

BEFORE AND AFTER BRONCHODILATOR STUDIES

A most practical application of pulmonary function testing is the determination of a course of therapy over and above the delineation of the nature and extent of a lesion.

Pulmonary function tests can be performed before and after bronchodilator therapy to determine the reversibility of lung dysfunction. The tests of pulmonary mechanics and of lung volumes are the usual parameters examined. The subject is given a normal battery of tests. Total lung capacity determinations done by He dilution or the open-circuit nitrogen method should be performed prior to bronchodilator administration to provide an accurate base line on which to judge the effects of the therapy.

A bronchodilator, usually isoproterenol or a preparation of similar action, can be administered by an aerosol generator or in conjunction with intermittent positive pressure breathing (IPPB). The extent of the therapy should be determined by the subject's requirements. For example, a known asthmatic patient may be given his regular bronchodilator between tests to determine that particular drug's effectiveness. Depending on the type of bronchodilator used and the means of administration, the therapy should last long enough to achieve the maximum effects. Most aerosolized bronchodilators begin taking effect on inhalation and continue for an indefinite period, usually at least an hour. If the bronchodilator is administered by IPPB, the "after" tests should be delayed for 5 to 10 minutes to allow for return of the blood gases to their normal values.

Reversibility of airway obstruction and improvement in flow rates is considered significant for increases of greater than 15%. Disease patterns involving the bronchial (and bronchiolar) musculature show the most pronounced change from "before" to "after." Uncomplicated asthma often shows improvements of greater than 50%. Moderate to severe chronic obstructive disease may fail to show any improvement and may even yield poorer results for the "after" tests because of the exertion of performing the forced expiratory tests several times. Since bronchodilators effect the greatest change in the pulmonary mechanics, repetition of the TLC tests is unnecessary. Any increase in vital capacity is usually at the expense of the previously increased residual volume. A common change is one in which the vital capacity increases only slightly, but the $FEF_{25\%-75\%}$ or $FEF_{200-1200}$ shows significant increase. This is caused by opening of previously constricted airways without notable increase in the actual volume of air moved by a forced expiratory maneuver.

EXERCISE TESTING

Performance of various pulmonary function tests, in conjunction with cardiac monitoring, provides an extension of the capability to diagnose cardiopulmonary disease or disability. Exercise increases cardiac output and pulmonary ventilation in response to the increased demands of muscles for oxygen delivery and CO_2 removal. Normal gas transfer requires efficiently operating lungs and chest bellows, effective pulmonary circulation with appropriately matching ventilation, and a cardiovascular system capable of meeting the metabolic demands of various tissues. In addition, a respiratory control mechanism capable of maintaining acid-base homeostasis by way of CO_2 clearance is necessary. Exercise testing ideally should provide information regarding the level of function for each link in the gas transport chain. For this reason, several parameters of cardiopulmonary function are measured during exercise. To quantify the level of function (or dysfunction), each parameter must be related to the *rate of work* being performed. Work is routinely expressed as the kilopound-meter (KPM), equivalent to the gravitational force acting on 1 kilogram as it is raised vertically 1 meter. Power output is also used to quantify the level of function and is expressed in kilopound-meters per minute (KPM/min) or in watts (600 KPM/min = 100 watts). Since there is a close relationship between power output and oxygen uptake, many of the variables measured during exercise can also be related easily to oxygen uptake. The unit of measurement for this purpose is the MET, which is defined as a multiple of the resting O_2 uptake (3.5 to 4.0 ml O_2/kg/min).

The parameters measured at various levels of exercise can be divided into two general categories: *invasive* and *noninvasive*.

Noninvasive measurements can be arranged into three groups:

1. ECG (electrocardiogram) to monitor heart rate and to determine the presence of arrhythmias and/or ischemia.
2. Expired ventilation and/or flow to monitor airflow limitation and pattern of Vt, f, and $\dot{V}e$ in relation to obstructive or restrictive processes.
3. Respired gas concentrations (O_2, CO_2, CO) to monitor oxygen uptake ($\dot{V}_{O_2}$), respiratory quotient (R), CO_2 production ($\dot{V}_{CO_2}$), end-tidal CO_2 (P_{ETCO_2}), and limitation to diffusion (D_{LCO}).

Invasive measurements can be arranged into two groups:

1. Systemic arterial puncture/catheterization to monitor Pa_{O_2}, Pa_{CO_2}, pH, Sa_{O_2}, HCO_3^-, blood lactate, mean arterial pressure (MAP), V_d/V_t in conjunction with the P_{ECO_2}, and the alveolar-arterial oxygen gradient (A-aDO_2).
2. Pulmonary arterial catheterization to monitor pulmonary artery pressure (PAP), pulmonary wedge pressure (PWP), mixed venous gas tensions, and cardiac output (CO).

Exercise testing is commonly performed using one, or both, of two basic regimens. The *progressive power output* test increases the work rate by a constant amount in steps of 1-minute intervals. The test is continued until the subject's maximum exercise level is attained or until a certain power output or heart rate is attained. A target heart rate of 85% of predicted maximum (according to age) is commonly used but may be unrealistic in patients with known or suspected ischemic heart disease. In the progressive power output test, steady state values for $\dot{V}_{O_2}$, $\dot{V}_{CO_2}$, and other parameters are not usually attained. To obtain steady state values, the *constant power output regimen* is used. Two to three submaximal power output levels are chosen, and the subject exercises at each level until a steady state of heart rate, O_2 uptake, and CO_2 production is attained. The subject then exercises for 2 minutes at this steady state at each level until the necessary gas collection or blood sampling is performed. Exercise at each power output is maintained for 5 to 8 minutes in this way.

Work or power output is quantified by exercising the subject on a treadmill or cycle ergometer. Each of these methods offers relative advantages. The treadmill approximates "normal" walking exercise. Adjustment of the speed and grade of incline of the treadmill varies the work load, but calculation of power output is complicated because the subject's body weight and walking pattern must be considered. The treadmill does allow maximal levels to be attained easily because of the large muscle groups involved in walking or jogging.

The cycle ergometer offers the most precise means of quantifying the work performed, since it exercises a sufficiently large group of muscles to induce cardiopulmonary stress, but at the same time eliminates the dependence of work rate on the subject's body weight (because the cycle supports the body). With cycle ergometers the work load can be changed quickly and easily by adding known resistances to the pedals. The subject's upper body is more stable than when walking, allowing blood sampling or catheterization to be easily performed. Other forms of exercise, such as stair-climbing or handgrip exercises, offer great difficulty in calculating the amount of work performed.

Ventilatory parameters during exercise ($\dot{V}_E$, Vt, f, etc.) can be measured with the same types of instruments as used in simple pulmonary function testing. The response frequency of spirometers must be considered since rapid breathing rates are commonly attained. Water-seal or dry rolling-seal spirometers (see Chapter 8) may not give adequate reproduction of ventilation at rapid rates. For totalized volumes, exhaled gas may be collected in a large volume bag (such as the Douglas bag) and then measured by emptying it into a large spirometer or through a gas meter. For most purposes, volume measurement by means of a pneumotach (see Chapter 8) and an integrating circuit offers many advantages. In instances where breath-by-breath measurement is required or where volume output must be processed together with the output of various gas analyzers, the pneumotach is quite suitable. The pneumotachometer may be affected by rapid temperature changes or condensation in the pneumotach tube, and these effects can limit its usefulness.

Analysis of $\dot{V}_{O_2}$ and $\dot{V}_{CO_2}$ require gas analyzers of suitable accuracy. In instances where concentrations are being measured in collected gas samples, slow response analyzers are adequate. When breath-by-breath analysis is required, rapid response analyzers are necessary. The infrared analyzer is commonly used for CO_2 as well as CO determinators (see Chapter 8). Because O_2 is usually analyzed from a sampling bag, a simple analyzer based on either the paramagnetic or polarographic principle may be used. For simultaneous, rapid analysis of several gases, the mass spectrometer is the instrument of choice. Mass spectrometers designed for clinical use such as exercise testing are currently being marketed.

Electrocardiographic monitoring is normally done with chest leads (V_5) to eliminate artifact caused by motion of the limbs. Sophisticated monitoring systems use a series of chest electrodes to allow selection of one of several lead combinations. Resuscitation equipment should be included as standard in every clinical exercise testing facility. Equipment should include a DC defibrillator (in addition to cardiac monitor), manual resuscitator with high oxygen delivery capability, airways, endotracheal tubes and laryngoscope, and drugs commonly provided for advanced cardiopulmonary resuscitation.

PULMONARY FUNCTION TESTING IN CHILDREN

Pulmonary function testing in children uses the same basic tests as are used in adults. Differences between adult and pediatric testing exist not only in the absolute dimensions of the developing pulmonary system but in two main areas concerned with the testing regimens themselves:

1. Newborns, infants, and very young children cannot strictly perform those tests that require and depend on subject cooperation.
2. Young children and adolescents may perform variably on those tests that are effort dependent or that require detailed instruction.

Tests of lung function in infants and very young children normally assess lung volumes and those mechanical factors that are not determined by the functional limits of the respiratory system. Inability to perform maximal efforts eliminates such parameters as **FVC** or **FEF**. Reasonable estimates of basic measurements, such as the vital capacity, can be made by compromise techniques, but the details are beyond the scope of this text and the reader is directed toward the bibliography at the end of this chapter.

Pulmonary function testing in children and adolescents is often directed toward diagnosis and evaluation of the disease states most common in pediatric subjects. These are (1) asthma, (2) cystic fibrosis, and (3) chest deformities.

The presence and severity of asthma in children is evaluated using a method similar to that used for testing the extent of reversible obstructive lung disease in adults.

1. *Lung volume measurements* (VC, TLC, RV, FRC, RV/TLC) provide information concerning hyperinflation (air trapping) particularly in acute asthmatic episodes.
2. *Flow measurements* (FEF_x, FEV_T, $FEV_{t\%}$, MEFV curves, PEFR) help to establish the extent of obstruction and determine the effect of bronchodilators. The PEFR (peak expiratory flow rate) can be particularly useful since it can be measured conveniently (at the

bedside with a portable peak flow meter) and provides serial measurements for planning and evaluating therapy. PEFR should be correlated with other flow measurements.

3. *Exercise testing* may be used to determine the presence of exercise-induced bronchospasm and to evaluate the effectiveness of particular therapeutic regimens.

The progression of lung function deterioration in children with *cystic fibrosis* is measured in a manner similar to that used in adults with chronic obstructive pulmonary disease (COPD).

1. *Lung volumes* (VC, FRC, RV, TLC, RV/TLC) provide data concerning air trapping.

2. *Flow measurements* (FEF_X, FEV_T, $FEV_t\%$, MEFV curves) assess the extent of obstruction caused by mucus plugging, bronchospasm, and edema.

3. *Arterial blood gases* provide information concerning the degree of respiratory insufficiency.

Chest deformities that are commonly evaluated by pulmonary function studies include kyphoscoliosis and pectus excavatum. In both cases, measurements include those parameters that are useful in assessing restrictive ventilatory patterns, such as lung volumes and D_{LCO}.

Normal values of lung function for children in all cases depend on height, sex, and age. Nomograms for lung volumes and various flow measurements for common parameters are included in the Appendix.

BEDSIDE TESTING

The determination of a course of therapy is one of the most common indications for pulmonary function studies. In many situations, these determinations must necessarily be performed at the bedside rather than under laboratory conditions. Evaluation of patients in the clinical setting involves three main types of pulmonary function tests: (1) ventilation, (2) pulmonary mechanics, and (3) matching of ventilation and blood flow.

Ventilation tests ($\dot{V}_E$, V_T, f, VC)

Basic ventilatory measurements are fundamental to the treatment of patients requiring continuous ventilatory assistance, those with impending ventilatory failure, or in the early stages of recovery from ventilatory failure. Ventilation tests correlate well with arterial blood gas studies in determining the type and duration of ventilatory assistance required for patients in acute ventilatory failure.

Pulmonary mechanics tests (FVC, FEV, FEF, PEFR, NIF)

Measurements of forced vital capacity and flow rates at the bedside provide a quantitative basis for therapy in obstructive airway processes, particularly asthma. Portable spirometers and pneumotachometers allow serial measurements, on a daily or even hourly basis, to assess the effectiveness of bronchodilators, respiratory therapy, or chest physical therapy.

Peak expiratory flow rates (PEFR), though used often, do not by themselves quantify the reversibility of obstruction since normal peak flows may be developed early in a forced expiration despite decreased FEV or FEF values. PEFR should be correlated with other flow measurements rather than used alone.

Negative inspiratory force (NIF) is measured by connection of a pressure manometer to an occluded airway and noting the maximum negative pressure that can be developed. The NIF is used in obtunded patients in whom the FVC cannot be obtained. Occlusion of the airway produces maximal values within 10 to 20 seconds, but may not be tolerated well by patients with unstable cardiovascular status. A vital capacity of 15 ml/kg requires development of approximately -20 cm H_2O, and this value is considered the minimum below which a patient usually will not be able to maintain adequate spontaneous ventilation over an extended period. Values greater than -80 cm H_2O are observed in healthy individuals, but negative pressures greater than -20 cm H_2O in obtunded patients have not been well correlated with specific vital capacities.

Ventilation/blood flow matching tests

Arterial blood gas analysis (see Chapter 6) is the most commonly used method of evaluating the adequacy of ventilation/blood flow matching.

Two techniques that have proved especially valuable in the clinical setting are the determinations of dead space (V_D/V_T ratio) and clinical shunt ($\dot{Q}s/\dot{Q}t$) (see Chapter 6). Shunt and dead space measurements may be performed on patients requiring continuous ventilatory assistance without interruption of the therapy. Serial measurements of shunt and dead space provide data concerning the progression of a patient's clinical status and allow for changes in the ventilator therapy appropriate for the patient's status. Simple measurement of the alveolar-arterial oxygen gradient ($A\text{-}aDO_2$) with the patient breathing 100% O_2 provides similar information in instances where the calculation of percent shunt may be unreliable, such as when the true a-v content difference cannot be measured. $A\text{-}aDO_2$ values of less than 250 mm Hg while breathing 100% oxygen are consistent with adequate matching of ventilation and perfusion to allow weaning from mechanical ventilation to be considered. Normal healthy adults show $A\text{-}aDO_2$s of 50 to 100 mm Hg while breathing pure oxygen.

Measurement of end-tidal CO_2 tension (P_{ETCO_2}), either by manual or automatic sampling, provides information similar to that obtained from the dead space measurement. Averaged end-tidal values may be used to calculate the V_D/V_T ratio if the arterial CO_2 tension is known, but may be inaccurate in the presence of severe $\dot{V}/\dot{Q}$ abnormalities.

Mechanical spirometers, such as the Wright respirometer (see Chapter 8), provide the most simple and portable means of measuring $\dot{V}_E$, V_T, and VC. Measurement of FVC, FEV_T, and FEF_X, is most easily accomplished by means of a portable electronic spirometer, using one of several flow-sensing transducer principles and integrating circuitry. Many available portable spirometers provide output including measured, predicted, and percent of predicted and can be adapted to provide hard-copy printout. PEFR can be measured by portable electronic spirometers or by mechanical flow-sensing devices such as the Wright-Peak flow meter. NIF is measured simply by connecting a manometer, calibrated in cm H_2O or mm Hg, to either an anatomically fitting face mask or a standard artificial airway connector. A means for rapidly occluding and reopening the airway must be provided.

SELECTED BIBLIOGRAPHY

Clinical spirometry: Recommendations of the Section on Pulmonary Function Testing, Committee on Pulmonary Physiology, American College of Chest Physicians, Dis. Chest **43**:214, 1963.

Comroe, J. H., Jr., Forster, R. E., Dubois, A. B., Briscoe, W. A., and Carlsen, E.: The lung: clinical physiology and pulmonary function tests, Chicago, 1962, Year Book Medical Publishers, Inc.

Comroe, J. H., Jr., and Nadel, J. A.: Current concepts: screening tests of pulmonary function, N. Engl. J. Med. **282**:1249, 1970.

Gandevia, B., and Hugh-Jones, P.: Terminology for measurements of ventilatory capacity: a report to the Thoracic Society, Thorax **12**:290, 1957.

Jones, N. L., Campbell, E. J. M., Edwards, R. H. T., and Robertson, W. G.: Clinical exercise testing, Philadelphia, 1975, W. B. Saunders Co.

Leiner, G. C., Abramowitz, S., and Small, M. J.: Pulmonary function testing in laboratories associated with residency training programs in pulmonary diseases, Am. Rev. Respir. Dis. **100**:240, 1969.

Light, R. W., Conrad, S. A., and George, R. B.: The one best test for evaluating the effects of bronchodilator therapy, Chest **72**:512, 1977.

Polgar, G., and Promadhat, V.: Pulmonary function testing in children, Philadelphia, 1971, W. B. Saunders Co.

Wasserman, K., and Whipp, B. J.: Exercise physiology in health and disease, Am. Rev. Respir. Dis. **112**:219, 1975.

Woolcock, A. J., Colman, M. H., and Blackburn, C. R. B.: Factors affecting normal values for ventilatory lung function, Am. Rev. Respir. Dis. **106**:692, 1972.

CHAPTER EIGHT

Pulmonary function testing equipment

Although many of the principles of pulmonary function testing that date back a hundred years are still in use, recent years have seen an astounding multiplication of devices for assessing the various parameters of pulmonary function. Testing by means of electronic as well as mechanical apparatus has proceeded toward a rather specialized technology. Nonetheless, complex testing procedures are common on a widespread basis.

Many of the tests that are a common part of testing regimens developed as a result of technical advances in regard to the respective testing device. This chapter enumerates and attempts to explain the principles of the more common pieces of hardware in current use, in terms of specific testing applications. Included are spirometers, bellows, respirometers, pneumotachs, gas analyzers, plethysmographs, and recording and output devices.

SPIROMETERS
Water-seal spirometers

For many years the basic tool in the determination of lung volumes and capacities and flow rates has been the water-seal spirometer. The water-seal spirometer consists of a large bell suspended in a container of water with the open end of the bell below the surface of the water (Fig. 8-1). A breathing system into and out of the interior of the bell allows for the addition or removal of accurate amounts of gas. Normally the subject breathes into and out of the spirometer and in so doing

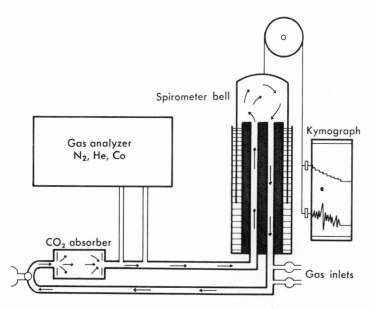

Fig. 8-1. Water-seal spirometer. Typical water-seal spirometer apparatus, including one-way breathing circuit, CO_2 remover, and recording kymograph (see text). (From Clinical spirometry, Braintree, Mass., Warren E. Collins, Inc.)

moves the bell a proportional distance. The movement of the bell can be used to mechanically manipulate a pen attached to a kymograph or to activate an electrical potentiometer to produce an output signal. The breathing system necessarily includes a CO_2 remover (soda lime) for rebreathing studies and separate inspiratory and expiratory circuits to eliminate dead space.

Water-seal spirometers are commonly used for the following tests:

1. Lung volumes and subdivisions (including RV and TLC when used with appropriate gas analyzers)
2. Ventilation (minute volume and tidal volume)
3. Diffusing capacity (with appropriate gas analyzers)
4. Pulmonary mechanics, including FVC, FEV_T, and

FEV$_T$%, inspiratory and expiratory flow rates, and MVV

The reliability of the water-seal spirometer depends on a number of factors. Primarily, the spirometer bell must be precisely counterweighted so that respiratory excursions are accurately reproduced. The resistance to movement (inertia) of the bell must be considered in calculating final results, especially in the case of timed vital capacities and flow rates. In systems in which the movement of the spirometer bell mechanically traces a spirogram, correction must be made for changes in temperature and saturation of expired gas. Units in which the bell activates a potentiometer are usually equipped

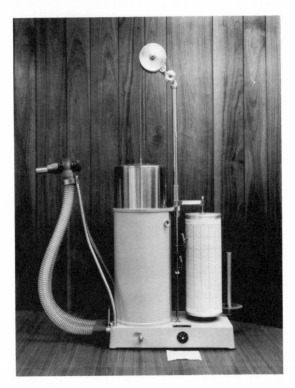

Fig. 8-2. Collins spirometer. Collins water-seal spirometer with counterweight pulley, kymograph, and breathing circuit. (Courtesy Warren E. Collins, Inc., Braintree, Mass.)

with signal corrections from ATPS to BTPS. Individual manufacturers will give specific details as to what corrections are
necessary and how they are to be made for their particular instruments.

Two water-seal spirometers are in common use. The Collins spirometer has been the basic tool of pulmonary function
testing for over a decade (Fig. 8-2). This water-seal spirometer
is available in a variety of sizes. The earlier models feature a 9-
or 13.5-liter bell, and the new modular unit features inter-
changeable 7- and 14-liter bells. The basic unit employs a bell
counterweighted by a pulley, with two recording pens and a
variable speed kymograph. One pen records respiratory excursions during inspiration as well as expiration, the other during
inspiration only, thus tracing accumulated volumes (minute
volume, MVV, etc.). The kymograph has speeds of 32, 160,
and 1920 mm/min, so that timed capacities can be conveniently recorded.

The Stead-Wells water-seal spirometer (Fig. 8-3) operates
on the basic principles just outlined, with the exception of
employing a lightweight plastic bell not counterweighted or
supported by pulleys. The Stead-Wells spirometer carries a
recording pen mounted against a variable speed kymograph,
but, unlike the Collins spirometer, inspiratory excursions
deflect the pen downward, and expiratory excursions deflect it
upward. The Collins spirometer traces the spirogram in an
inverted manner because of the pulley-driven recording pens.
The Stead-Wells spirometer offers less inertia and hence is
somewhat more suitable for those tests measuring flow rates
during the early part of an FEV maneuver, such as the
$FEF_{200-1200}$.

Dry rolling-seal spirometers

One of the more recent innovations in spirometry is the dry
rolling-seal spirometer. A typical unit consists of a piston in a
cylinder, which is supported by a rod resting on frictionless
bearings (Fig. 8-4). The piston is coupled to the cylinder wall
by a plastic seal that rolls on itself rather than sliding. The

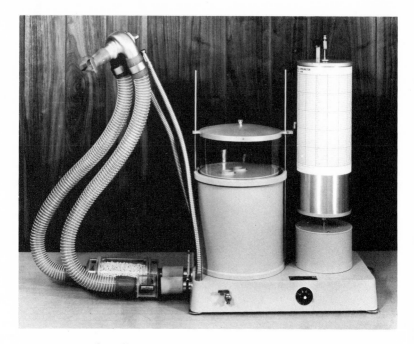

Fig. 8-3. Stead-Wells spirometer. Stead-Wells spirometer, with lightweight, noncounterweighted bell, kymograph, and breathing circuit. (Courtesy Warren E. Collins, Inc., Braintree, Mass.)

volume of the piston/cylinder combination is usually 10 to 12 liters, but the piston is of large enough diameter so that excursions of just a few inches produce large volume changes. The piston is normally lightweight aluminum so that there is little inertia or mechanical resistance.

The dry-seal spirometer is suitable for the same tests as the water-seal spirometers:

1. Lung volumes
2. Ventilation
3. Diffusing capacity
4. Pulmonary mechanics

Some dry rolling-seal spirometers employ mechanically driven graphing devices in which the piston itself moves a

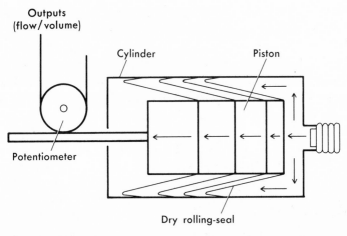

Fig. 8-4. Dry rolling-seal spirometer. Cutaway view of the main components of a typical dry rolling-seal spirometer. The figure gives an exaggerated view of the rolling-seal, which actually fits closely between the piston and cylinder wall. The piston has a large surface area, so that its horizontal movement is kept at a minimum. This allows recording of normal and forced respiratory excursions with only a small amount of mechanical movement and hence little mechanical resistance. The piston rides on a rod that activates an electrical potentiometer. The rotational movement of the potentiometer is translated into output signals of flow and volume. (From Form 370, Madison, Wis., Ohio Medical Products.)

pen. Most, however, have a potentiometer that is activated by the movement of the piston to provide an electrical output for volume and flow. Since the dry-seal spirometer is so readily adapted to producing electrical outputs for both volume and flow, most of the currently available systems have analog function computers with digital readouts and hard-copy recorders either built in or available in modular form. Since the dry-seal spirometer travels in a horizontal plane, there is no need for counterbalancing or correction factors. Some systems feature electronic corrections for spirometer resistance, temperature, saturation, and gas viscosity, thus eliminating a number of time-consuming calculations. One-way circuits and CO_2 removers are available, so that dry-seal spirometers can be used for rebreathing tests in the same way as water-seal spirometers.

Dry rolling-seal spirometers, employing the basic design just outlined, are available from several manufacturers. Most include elctronic BTPS corrections and preset calibration signals for both flow and volume signals. The latter allow for fast checks of the integrity of the output signals from the spirometer. Most such units are compatible with analog computers that accept flow and volume input, as well as strip and chart recorders (pp. 127 to 131).

Bellows spirometers

A third type of spirometer is the bellows or wedge bellows, which consists of a collapsible bellows that folds or unfolds in

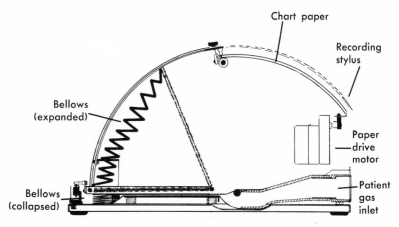

Fig. 8-5. Wedge bellows spirometer. Cross-sectional diagram of a wedge bellows spirometer. The fanlike movements of the wedge bellows produce mechanical movement, which is usually translated directly to the recording device. Some manufacturers suspend the bellows so that the primary movement is in a horizontal rather than vertical direction; large wedge bellows designed in this manner offer relatively little mechanical resistance and are comparable to dry-seal or water-seal spirometers in accuracy and linearity. (Adapted from Vitalograph Medical Instrumentation, Product Brochure, Lenexa, Ka., 1976.)

response to breathing excursions. The wedge bellows design is more common than conventional bellows because it offers less mechanical resistance. The wedge bellows opens and closes somewhat like a fan (Fig. 8-5). Since one side of the bellows remains stationary, the other side moves with a pivotal motion around an axis through the fixed side, and this displacement of the bellows by a volume of gas is transmitted to a mechanical recording device. The recording chart is arranged to move at a fixed speed under the pen and thus traces a spirogram.

The wedge bellows (and conventional bellows) is suitable for measurement of the vital capacity and some of its subdivisions, timed vital capacities, and pulmonary mechanics, including inspiratory/expiratory flow rates and MVV. The most common disadvantage of the wedge bellows design is inaccuracy resulting from the inertia or resistance of the bellows. A number of manufacturers have introduced designs that eliminate most of the mechanical resistance, but deviations tend to occur at extremes of flow or volume change. Corrections for BTPS must be made or included in the scale of the recording chart paper.

Wright respirometer

A fourth type of basic spirometer is the Wright respirometer, which consists of a vane connected to a series of gears such that gas flowing through the body of the instrument rotates the vane and registers a volume (Fig. 8-6). This type of respirometer is suitable for measurement of lung volumes such as the vital capacity and ideal for ventilation tests such as tidal volume and minute volume. The wright respirometer can be used to measure volumes at flows between 3 and 300 L/min. At flows above 300 L/min the vane is subject to distortion and therefore should not be used to measure FVC when the subject is capable of flows greater than 300 L/min. At flows less than 3 L/min the inertia of the vane/gear system causes erroneous measurements. The special advantage of the respirometer is its compact size and practicality in the bedside set-

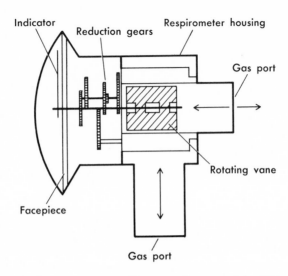

Fig. 8-6. Wright respirometer. Cutaway diagram of the Wright respirometer. A large bladed rotating vane mounted on jeweled bearings drives reduction gears connected to the main indicator arm. Two gas ports allow measurements of totalized volume, either inspiratory or expiratory, depending on the port to which connection is made. Not pictured is a small indicator arm, which marks volumes larger than 1 liter on the facepiece; also omitted are instrument controls for engaging or disengaging the vane and for resetting the indicators to zero. (From The British Oxygen Co., Ltd. Operating Instructions, Wright Respirometer, print No. 630207, Issue 3:6, Aug., 1971.)

ting. The respirometer registers tenths of liters up to 1 liter on the large scale and liters up to 100 liters on the small scale, which makes it ideal for measuring volumes over longer periods. Volumes greater than 1 liter sometimes make it difficult to read the small scale.

PNEUMOTACHS

In contrast to mechanical spirometers of the water-seal, dry rolling-seal, or bellows types is the pneumotach. Pneumotachs utilize various physical properties to produce an electrical output that can be integrated for measurement of volumes and flows. Although a wide variety of types of pneumotachs are presently available, three basic designs are commonly used.

The first of these is a tube through which laminar airflow is possible. Within the tube, in the path of the gas flow, is a resistive element that allows gas to flow through it but causes a pressure drop. The pressure differential is measured by means of sensitive pressure transducers, which convert the differential to a signal (Fig. 8-7). The resistive element is usually a screen or similar device that allows gas to flow through without undue back pressure while at the same time causing a significant pressure drop to produce a signal. Since the diameter and length of the tube at the resistive element remain fixed, the pressure difference is proportional to the flow. The signal from the pressure transducers can be electronically integrated for a given interval to derive a volume measurement.

The second most common type of pneumotach is that which is based on the cooling effect of gas flow. A heated element (usually a platinum wire) is situated in a tube. Gas flow past the element causes a temperature drop so that more current is required to maintain the preset temperature of the element. The amount of current needed to maintain the temperature is proportional to the magnitude of the gas flow. The heated element is usually of very small mass so that slight changes in gas flow can be detected. (Temperature change occurs more rapidly in objects of small mass.) The signal is applied to an integrator circuit as with the pressure transducer pneumotach to derive volume measurements.

A third type of flow sensing instrument is designed according to the principle of vortex shedding. A flow tube is constructed with struts placed in the airstream so that gas flowing over the struts is broken up into waves called *vortices*. An ultrasonic crystal downstream of the strut transmits high frequency sound waves through the turbulent gas flow to a receiving crystal on the opposite side (Fig. 8-8). The size of the strut and flow tube determine the size of the vortices and allow the device to be calibrated so that each vortex passing

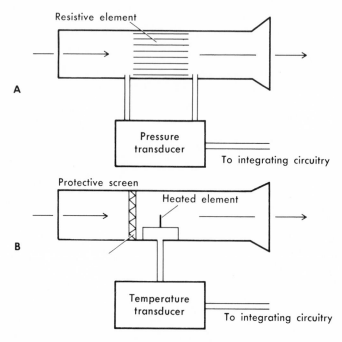

Fig. 8-7. Two conventional pneumotachs. **A,** Pressure-drop type of pneumotach, in which a resistive element causes a pressure drop proportional to the flow of gas through the tube. Sensitive pressure transducers monitor the pressure before and after the resistive element and convert the differential into a signal that varies as the flow changes. The volume passing through the pneumotach can be calculated by integrating the flow over the time interval for which the flow occurred; this is done by an electronic integrating circuit. **B,** A heat transfer type of pneumotach in which a heated element of small mass responds to gas flow by heat loss. As the element cools, a greater current is needed to maintain a constant temperature; the current change is proportional to gas flow, and a continuous signal is supplied to an integrating circuit as for the pressure drop pneumotach.

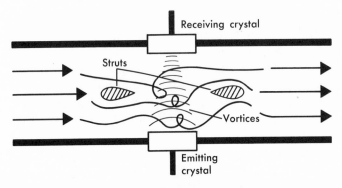

Fig. 8-8. Ultrasonic flow sensor. A beam of ultrasonic waves is emitted by one crystal and received by another crystal on the opposite side of the flow tube. Gas flowing in streamlines passes over struts in the tube and forms vortices. This is called *vortex shedding* and changes the frequency of the transmitted ultrasound waves. Appropriate signals are processed electronically to derive flow and volume measurements. Flow (and volume) can be measured for gas moving in either direction.

through the ultrasonic beam produces a pulse. The number of pulses are proportional to flow and, when combined with integrating circuitry, provide measurement of volumes. The ultrasonic pneumotach is relatively insensitive to gas composition, temperature, or humidity, although accumulation of moisture on the struts or ultrasonic transducers can cause erroneous readings.

Most of the pneumotachs available are designed on one of these three basic principles. Several instruments, however, use a rotating vane, much like that in the Wright respirometer, to measure flow rates. Normally these mechanical pneumotachs measure only flow, since there is no electrical output to be applied to an integrating circuit. Some mechanical pneumotachs are adapted to produce an output signal by means of a light-chopping vane rotating over a series of photocells, which produce a signal proportional to the velocity of the vane.

Pneumotachs with suitable electrical outputs can be used for the following measurements:

1. Lung volumes (with appropriate integrating circuitry), including TLC and RV (with gas analyzers)
2. Ventilation, including tidal volume and minute volume
3. Distribution (with appropriate gas analyzers)
4. Pulmonary mechanics, including MVV, FEV_T, $FEV_{T\%}$, and flow rates

Pulmonary function testing with the pneumotach offers numerous advantages over classic spirometry setups. The most obvious of these is the ability to do precise testing with lightweight compact units. The fact that a signal is generated without the mechanical action of a spirometer or bellows allows for more direct processing of information. Strip chart or X-Y recorders can be directly connected to the basic pneumotach/calculator setup to produce hard-copy data along with digital readout of test results.

The disadvantages of the pneumotach-type testing units should not be overlooked. All instruments using a pneumotach as the basic measuring device are not created equal. Pneumotachography is based on the assumption that a certain airflow will generate a proportional signal. However, at extremes of flow (low or high) the signal generated becomes nonproportional, or nonlinear. This is true of almost every type of pneumotach. Many systems use two pneumotachs, one for high flows as in forced breathing and one for low flows as in tidal volume excursions. The signal from this type of system is more linear across the range of the pneumotach because the range itself is reduced. Most units "linearize" the signal electronically before any parameters are measured so that the values will be accurate to within acceptable limits. Other corrections, such as converting results to BTPS, can be done easily by electronic means. Most units that utilize resistive elements to cause a pressure differential include a means of heating the element to above body temperature so as to avoid deviations resulting from condensation of water in the element.

The final results from any measurement done with a pneumotach are only as accurate as the circuitry that converts the primary signal to actual readout values or hard-copy tracing. Those pulmonary function parameters that are measured on a time base (FEV_T, MVV, $FEF_{200-1200}$, etc.) require precise timing mechanisms as well as volume or flow measurements. The most common timing mechanism in pneumotachography is the initiation of a specific test interval by a minimum flow or pressure change. Recording flow or volume on a time base begins when the flow generated through the pneumotach has reached a threshold limit, usually around 0.2 L/sec. Instruments that initiate timing in response to pressure change usually have a similar threshold that must be achieved to begin recording the input signal. Standards for spirometers and flow-sensing devices according to individual tests are included in the Appendix.

PULMONARY GAS ANALYZERS

The determination of the composition of pulmonary gases is an integral part of tests for distribution of inspired gas, FRC, RV, and diffusion.

The most commonly used gas analyzer is that which determines the concentration of nitrogen in respired gas; the single breath and 7-minute nitrogen distribution, as well as the open-circuit method of determining the RV (Chapter 1), require N_2 analyzers. A common N_2 analyzer is the Giesler tube-type ionizer (Fig. 8-9). This instrument consists of a needle valve that samples the desired gas, an enclosed ionization chamber with two electrodes, and a photocell. A vacuum pump maintains a constant pressure in the ionization chamber by bleeding gas through the needle valve. When a current is supplied to the electrodes, the nitrogen between them is ionized and emits light. This light, after being filtered, is collected by a phototube. The intensity of the light is directly related to the concentration of N_2 in the sample, provided that the current, distance between electrodes, and pressure remain constant. The phototube converts the light signal into an electrical signal, which is linearized and then can be used as input

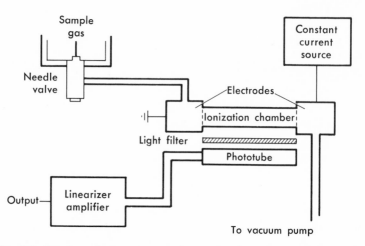

Fig. 8-9. Giesler tube type gas analyzer. Giesler tube gas analyzer as is commonly used for nitrogen analysis. A vacuum pump draws a gas sample into an ionization chamber, where the ionized gas emits light (all except the desired gas is filtered), which is monitored by a phototube. The phototube transmits a signal proportional to the intensity of the light, and the signal allows rapid gas analysis. (From Application note AN 729, San Diego, Calif., 1973, Hewlett-Packard.)

to an appropriate meter or computing circuit. The signal from the N_2 analyzer can be combined with the volume signal from electronic units to provide instantaneous, or breath-by-breath, measurements of nitrogen volumes as necessary for open-circuit determinations of the FRC. An older method of measuring the FRC by the open-circuit method depended on measuring the concentration of N_2 in a large volume of expired gas (washed out) in a Tissot spirometer. This method was susceptible to error because of the measurement of a small concentration of N_2 in a large volume. The accumulation of breath-by-breath measurements has obviated this difficulty, since the FRC calculation is not dependent on a single measurement.

The calculation of FRC and residual volume by the closed-circuit technique requires a helium analyzer or catharometer.

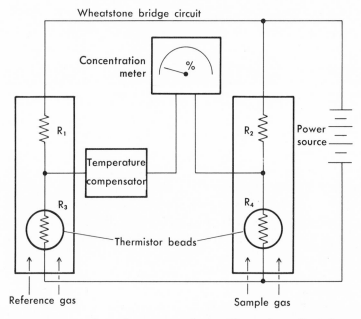

Fig. 8-10. Thermal conductivity analyzer. Thermal conductivity gas analyzer such as is used for analysis of CO_2 and He. Two thermistor beads (temperature-sensitive electrical resistors) are connected in a wheatstone bridge circuit. When the thermistors are subjected to the same gas, their electrical resistance decreases equally and the concentration meter registers zero (by calibration). When the sample gas is applied to the sample thermistor, R_4 in this case, and the reference thermistor submitted to the reference gas, a potential occurs and deflects the concentration meter by a proportionate amount. (From Life systems operations instruction manual, Model LS114-5, Riverside, Calif., 1973, Bourns, Inc.)

The catharometer measures the concentration of helium in the sample gas by means of a thermal conductivity sensing unit (Fig. 8-10). Two glass-coated thermistor beads serve as sensing elements connected by a wheatstone bridge circuit. The sensors change temperature and hence electrical resistance as a function of the molecular weight of the gases surrounding them. One bead serves as a reference, so that a difference in the concentration of gases at the two sensors can be detected because of the differences in heat conducted away at either of the sensors. Since the closed-cicuit technique mixes only a small volume of He in the larger volume of the lungs and breathing system (Chapter 1), the catharometer usually is calibrated for measuring small fractional concentrations of He. The small necessary range allows for good linearity and sensitivity.

Perhaps the most sophisticated means of measuring the concentrations of respiratory gases is the mass spectrometer. A sample of gas is drawn into a capillary tube by a vacuum pump, which reduces simultaneously the pressure to a preset level. An electron beam ionizes the sample gases, which are directed into a beam by an electrostatic lens. As the beam passes through a magnetic field, the ions of the various constit-

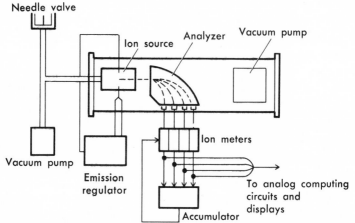

Fig. 8-11. Mass spectrometer. A mass spectrometer in which respiratory gases are analyzed thus: a vacuum pump draws a small sample of gas into an ionizing chamber, where a current sufficient to ionize the desired gases is supplied; a magnetic analyzer separates the ion beam into constituent gases; the separated beams are collected by distinct ion meters, and the relative concentration of each gas is determined in opposition to a reference gas. These parameters emerge as signals to computing and display circuits. (From advertising brochure for Model 1100, Medical gas analyzer, Pomona, Calif., Perkin-Elmer Medical Instruments.)

uent gases separate according to their specific mass and electrical charge (Fig. 8-11). Ion collectors gather the various ions and amplify their charges into a usable signal for monitoring or analog computations. Analysis of the composition of a gas mixture on a breath-by-breath basis offers the possibility of performing several different tests requiring gas analysis with the same measuring device, as well as in vivo monitoring of respiratory gases. Although mass spectrometers allow gas analysis for such various tests as N_2 washout or CO diffusing capacity with a single analyzer, their relative cost is somewhat prohibitive.

A number of respiratory gas analyzers are based on the principle of infrared absorption to measure gas concentrations. This techique is most often used in CO analyzers for $D_{L_{CO}}$ tests. Two beams of infrared radiation pass through two parallel cells, one of which contains gas to be sampled, the other containing a comparison gas. The two beams converge on a single infrared detector (Fig. 8-12). Between the test cells and the infrared source an interrupter alternates the beams to the cells. When the test gas and comparison gas are the same concentration, the radiation reaching the detector is constant; but when the sample gas is introduced, the amount of radiation reaching the detector varies in a rhythmic fashion. This causes a vibration in the detector that is translated into a signal proportional to the difference between the two beams. This type of system is readily adaptable to measurements involving small changes in gas concentrations such as those necessary in tests of diffusing capacity.

Measurements of aterial blood gases routinely include determination of P_{O_2}, P_{CO_2}, and pH.

The P_{O_2} *electrode* produces a current at a constant voltage that is proportional to the oxygen tension to which the electrode is exposed. This current is a result of the flow of electrons produced by the reduction of O_2 at the cathode according to the equation:

$$O_2 + 2H_2O + 4e^- \rightarrow 4OH^-$$

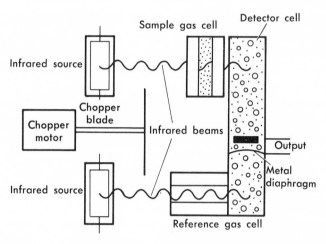

Fig. 8-12. Infrared absorption gas analyzer. Essential components of an infrared gas analyzer, such as is used for determination of CO concentrations. Infrared sources emit beams that pass through parallel cells, one containing a reference gas and the other the sample gas to be analyzed. A rotating blade "chops" the infrared beams in a rhythmic fashion so that when both the reference and sample cells contain the same gas, there is no variation in the radiation reaching either half of the detector cell. When the sample gas is introduced, differing amounts of radiation reach the two halves of the detector cell, causing the diaphragm separating the compartments of the detector to oscillate. This oscillation is transmitted into a signal proportional to the difference in gas concentrations. The infrared analyzer is thus ideal for determination of small concentration changes in gas samples. (From Medical gas analyzer LB-2: operating instructions, FM-149997-301, Schiller Park, Ill., 1972, Beckman Instruments, Inc.)

Each O_2 molecule can take up 4 electrons, and the greater the number of O_2 molecules present (P_{O_2}), the greater the current. The cathode of the electrode is covered by a membrane that is permeable to gases but not to other contaminates or ions (Fig. 8-13). Electrons are provided by a silver–silver chloride anode. A P_{O_2} electrolyte is enclosed in a reserve chamber around the anode and supplied to the tip by an annular capillary tube.

The P_{CO_2} electrode measures P_{CO_2} potentiometrically by an adaptation of a pH measurement. A combined pH glass and reference electrode is in contact with a solution behind a gas permeable membrane. CO_2 diffuses across the membrane in both directions as partial pressure changes, causing equilibration between the electrolyte and the sample. CO_2 is hydrated in the electrolyte according to the equation:

$$CO_2 + H_2O \leftrightarrow H_2CO_3 \leftrightarrow H^+ + HCO_3^-$$

The change in H^+ concentration is proportional to change in P_{CO_2}. The electrode senses the change in P_{CO_2} as a change in pH of the electrolyte and develops a voltage that is exponentially related to P_{CO_2}, so that a ten-fold increase in P_{CO_2} is approximately equal to a decrease of one pH unit (Fig. 8-13).

The glass pH electrode contains a solution of constant pH on one side of the glass membrane. The solution whose pH is to be measured is brought into contact with the other side of the pH-sensitive glass (Fig. 8-13). The difference in pH on either side causes a potential difference, or voltage. To measure this potential two half-cells are used: one for the constant solution and one for the unknown solution. The constant solution half-cell is usually a silver–silver chloride wire. The external half-cell in the unknown solution is usually a saturated calomel electrode and is called the *reference electrode*. These half-cells are connected to a millivolt display that is simply calibrated in pH units. The voltage difference between the two electrodes is proportional to the pH difference of the solutions. Since the pH of one solution is constant, the developed potential is a measure of the pH of the unknown solution.

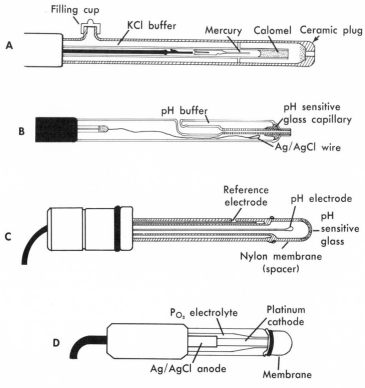

Fig. 8-13. For legend see opposite page.

PLETHYSMOGRAPHS

Whole-body plethysmography is a relatively recent addition to the battery of pulmonary function tests. The plethysmograph is used mainly for measurement of the thoracic gas volume (Chapter 1) and airway resistance (Chapter 3). Fundamental to both of these tests are measurements of flow rates, mouth pressures, and plethysmograph box pressure. Thus three basic measuring devices are necessary: a pneumotach for flows, a shutter apparatus for mouth pressures, and an air-

Fig. 8-13. pH, P_{CO_2}, and P_{O_2} electrodes. **A,** The reference pH electrode contains a sealed-in potassium chloride buffer and a porous ceramic plug that allow electrical contact to the exterior; the reference wire develops a constant potential. **B,** The pH measuring electrode contains buffer and a silver/silver chloride wire. A thin capillary tube constructed of pH-sensitive glass allows a potential to develop, which varies with the pH of the solution in the capillary. The difference between the variable potential and the constant potential of the reference electrode indicates the pH of the sample. **C,** The P_{CO_2} (Severinghaus) electrode is an adaptation of the pH electrode. The pH electrode contains a sealed-in buffer while the reference electrode is the other half-cell and is in communication with a P_{CO_2} electrolyte of aqueous bicarbonate. The entire glass electrode is encased in a Lucite jacket (not shown) containing the electrolyte and capped with a Teflon membrane that is permeable to CO_2. A nylon membrane covers the tip of the glass electrode to act as a spacer to keep electrolyte in contact with the pH-sensitive glass. CO_2 diffuses through the Teflon membrane, dissolves in the electrolyte, and alters the pH. The pH change is displayed as partial pressure of CO_2. **D,** The P_{O_2} electrode contains a platinum cathode and a silver/silver chloride anode. The tip is protected by a polyethylene or polypropylene membrane, which allows O_2 to diffuse. O_2 migrates to the cathode, which has a slightly negative charge or voltage. The oxygen is reduced by picking up free electrons that have come from the silver/silver chloride anode through the phosphate/potassium chloride buffer. Changes in the voltage result from changes in the amount of O_2 dissolved in the electrolyte, and this reflects P_{O_2}. A voltmeter measures the amount of change and registers it as partial pressure of oxygen.

---

tight body box for chamber pressures (Fig. 8-14). The pneumotach must have good linearity over the range used (0 to 2 L/sec) for both spontaneous breathing and panting. The mouth shutter, or interrupter, is usually coupled to the pneumotach so that obturation of the flow can be electronically initiated either at end-expiration or end-inspiration. In sequence, the chamber pressure and flow are measured and displayed either on an X-Y recorder or a storage oscilloscope.

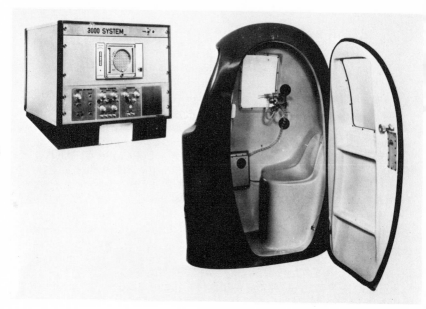

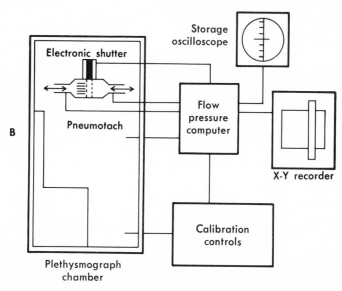

Fig. 8-14. Body plethysmograph. A, Typical plethysmograph setup. B, Diagram of plethysmograph components: low flow range pneumotach equipped with automatic shutter, airtight body box, interfacing computer for analysis of flow and pressure signals, storage oscilloscope and X-Y recorder to receive flow pressure output, and calibration controls for temperature compensation and automatic zeroing of flow and pressure channels. (A courtesy Ohio Medical Products, Division of Airco, Inc., Madison, Wis.)

Then the mouth pressure and chamber are measured simultaneously and recorded so that the true alveolar pressure can be derived.

A recent innovation in plethysmography has been the development of a volume plethymograph, in distinction to the pressure monitoring variety. The volume plethysmograph measures volume change, rather than pressure change, in the box by attachment to the box of either a mechanical (bellows) or electronic volume registering device. The volume change of the plethysmograph can be related directly to changes in alveolar volume. An advantage of the volume plethysmograph is that the body box need not be as rigorously airtight since sensitive pressure measurements are obviated.

The plethysmograph technique must take into account the fact that accurate measurements of chamber pressure include corrections or compensation for temperature and saturation changes caused by the respirations of the test subject.

Plethysmograph systems are available from several manufacturers. Most feature built-in calibration controls and are designed to allow subject comfort so that tests can be carried out quickly and without strain.

RECORDING AND OUTPUT DEVICES

An integral part of pulmonary function testing is the recording of spirograms, the various distribution and ventilation tests, and direct readout of values in digital form. From its inception, pulmonary function testing has concerned itself with the spirogram. The kymograph, a rotating drum carrying chart paper, was the initial instrument for producing a hard-copy record of respiratory movements (Fig. 8-2). A kymograph is a mechanical recorder in the strictest sense of the word, and normally corrections for BTPS must be made. Calibrated chart paper eliminates some corrections, but inherent factors such as mechanical resistance must be taken into account. Several of the most commonly used spirometers incorporate the kymograph recording system. Closely akin to the kymograph are those instruments that use mechanical recording on an X-Y type of graph. A constant speed motor provides movement along the time axis (X), and a bellows or spirometer provides the volume (Y) input. This principle is utilized in most wedge-bellows types of spirometers and in some rolling-seal spirometers. The same restrictions of mechanical resistance apply to these devices as were mentioned for the kymograph, except that in these the recording usually moves in a horizontal plane.

The obvious successor to a mechanical X-Y recorder has been the electronic X-Y recorder. In this instance a two-axis recorder receives electrical input in the form of a signal. The signal drives a small motor that controls the pen movement (Fig. 8-15). The advantage of this type of instrument is that several tests can be recorded by supplying an appropriate input signal, rather than simply a spirogram. The signal generated by a simple pneumotach or analog computing device can be recorded in spirographic form. Gas analyzers coupled to such an instrument allow easy recording of tests such as the single- and multiple-breath nitrogen washout. The electronic recorder is easy to calibrate; normally a small adjustment of the input signal is all that is required. Many recorders feature a third dimension for hard-copy recording in the form of superimposed time measurements, when the main input is not graphed on a time base. For instance, a flow-volume loop plots flow on the vertical axis and volume on the horizontal axis; an X-Y-T recorder can interpose time marks (tics) on the original tracing, thus allowing timed volumes to be obtained from the same tracing. Most electronic recorders have variable sensitivity on both axes, which allows for greater accuracy than a mechanical tracing. Systems equipped with digital readouts as well as an electronic recorder allow for easy comparisons of measured values and the spirogram.

Automated data collection, handling, and processing are becoming increasingly familiar in pulmonary function testing. Analog inputs from spirometers, pneumotachs, gas analyzers, plethysmographs, and blood gas analyzers can all be routed to a microprocessor or "true" computer by means of an analog-to-

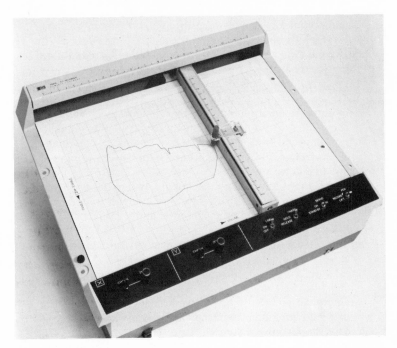

Fig. 8-15. X-Y recorder. An X-Y recorder capable of accepting flow and volume inputs and graphing either against a time base, or plotting flow against volume directly. (Courtesy Hewlett-Packard, San Diego, Calif.)

digital converter. (The boxed material on p. 130 lists terms commonly associated with automated data handling.) Signals can be stored, processed, compared, analyzed, and converted into a hard-copy printout in a matter of seconds. Tests that plot one variable against another such as $FEF_{25\%-75\%}$ (volume versus time) lend themselves to automated recording, since their precise measurement is largely a mathematical function. Comparison of a measured value to that which is predicted from a regression equation in done easily with a computer or microprocessor.

Analysis of a battery of test results to produce a differential diagnosis can only be as accurate as the program itself. Quali-

Terms commonly used in automated data handling

Analog input Electronic signal from a spirometer, gas analyzer, plethysmograph, or pneumotach

A/D convertor Analog-to-digital converter; changes electronic signals into computer language

Bit A unit of binary input (zero or nonzero)

Byte Approximately eight bits

Computer An electronic device that is centrally located and is capable of performing high speed calculations and assembling and storing information in a memory; computers can correlate and cross-reference by means of a logic or processor unit

CRT A control terminal consisting of a typewriter keyboard and viewing screen that allows the operator to manually supply information to the computer and to initiate and terminate procedures

Floppy disc A soft plastic disc with magnetic surface for storage of data and programs for rapid retrieval

Hardware The electromechanical devices comprising the computer and memory

Memory An electronic or mechanical device used to store data and programs; types of memory include magnetic core, floppy disc, magnetic tape, and tape casettes; the amount of information that can be stored is described in bits, each of which approximates one character; memory size is usually classified in *K*, thousands of bits, or *mega*, millions of bits

Microprocessor An electronic unit that is hardwired or contained on *chips*; microprocessors usually have fixed programs, perform calculations, do some assembly, and have a limited storage or memory

On-line A descriptive term denoting a direct connection between the testing instrument and the computer

Plotter An electromechanical device that converts digital outputs into tracings

Printer An electromechanical device that reports data in hard-copy form on paper

Real time A descriptive term denoting direct user response by the computer

Shared time A descriptive term denoting a computer with multiple users, working one at a time; the most sophisticated systems use a combination of real-time and shared-time modes

Software All programs including those that control computer functions and those that process input data

Word A specified number of bits

tative input, such as patient history, is not handled as readily as simple analog signals. Some analog inputs must be treated "qualitatively," and thus cannot be processed automatically. For example, the determination of the onset of Phase IV during the single-breath nitrogen test shows great variability among observers and can only be determined automatically when a sufficiently large memory is used to record and store enough "points" on the curve. Memory recording of curves does offer a good solution to the problems of mechanical resistance in either the input device (spirometer, etc.) or the output device (X-Y recorder, etc.). *Slewing* or overshoot (and undershoot) occurs when a mechanical pen fails to accurately produce a tracing representative of the true curve because of its own inertia or momentum. This normally occurs during maneuvers that are recorded rapidly, such as flow-volume curves. The problem of slewing is eliminated by storing the tracing as a large number of points in the memory and then plotting them afterwards at a slower speed.

Automated data handling can provide rapid and accurate recording of test parameters and allows technician attention to be directed toward patient effort and reproducibility of results. Programs that do not allow easy repetition of test maneuvers or restructuring of test sequence can affect the reproducibility of the values obtained.

SELECTED BIBLIOGRAPHY

Bartels, H., Bucheri, E., Heitz, C. W., Rodewald, G., and Schwab, M.: Methods in pulmonary physiology, translated by J. M. Workman, New York, 1963, Hafner Publishing Co.

Comroe, J. H., Jr., editor: Methods in medical research, vol. II, Pulmonary function tests, Chicago, 1950, Year Book Medical Publishers, Inc.

Finucane, K. E., Egan, B. R., and Dawson, S. V.: Linearity and frequency response of pneumotachographs, J. Appl. Physiol. **32:**1, 1972.

Fitzgerald, M. X., Smith, A. A., and Gaensler, E. A.: Evaluation of electronic spirometers, N. Engl. J. Med. **289:**1283, 1973.

Fry, D. L., Hyatt, R. E., McCall, C. B., and Mallos, A. S.: Evaluation of three types of respiratory flow meters, J. Appl. Physiol. **10:**210, 1957.

Grenvik, A., Hedstrand, U., and Sjorgen, H.: Problems in pneumotachography, Acta Anaesth. Scand. **10:**147, 1968.

Kory, R. C., and Hamilton, L. H.: Evaluation of spirometers used in pulmonary function studies, Am. Rev. Respir. Dis. **87:**288, 1963.

Smith, J. R., and Kory, R. C.: Laboratory aids in investigating pulmonary diseases. In Baum, G. L., editor: Textbook of pulmonary diseases, Boston, 1965, Little, Brown & Co.

Wells, H. S., Stead, W. W., Rossing, T. D., and Ognanovich, J.: Accuracy of an improved spirometer for recording fast breathing, J. Appl. Physiol. 14:451, 1959.

Wever, A. M. J., Britton, M. B., and Hughes, D. D. T.: Evaluation of two spirometers, Chest 70:244, 1976.

Wood, M.: Product analysis: pulmonary function analyzers for mass screening, Respir. Therapy 4:53, 1973.

Appendix

TYPICAL VALUES FOR PULMONARY FUNCTION TESTS (values are for a healthy young man, 1.7 m² body surface area)

TEST	VALUE
Lung volumes (BTPS)	
IC	3600 ml
ERV	1200 ml
VC	4800 ml
RV	1200 ml
FRC	2400 ml
TGV	2400 ml
TLC	6000 ml
(RV/TLC) × 100	20%
Ventilation (BTPS)	
V_T	500 ml
f	12 breaths/min
$\dot{V}_E$	6 L/min
V_D	150 ml
$\dot{V}_A$	4200 ml/min
Pulmonary mechanics	
FVC	4800 ml
$FEV_{0.5\%}$	60%
$FEV_{1.0\%}$	83%
$FEV_{2.0\%}$	94%
$FEV_{3.0\%}$	97%
$FEF_{200-1200}$	6 L/sec
$FEF_{25\%-75\%}$	4.7 L/sec
MVV	170 L/min
C_L	0.2 L/cm H_2O
C_{LT}	0.1 L/cm H_2O
Airway resistance (R_{aw})	1.6 cm H_2O/L/sec

Distribution

Single-breath N_2	Less than 1.5% N_2
Seven-minute N_2	Less than 2.5% N_2
IDI (ideal lung = 1.0)	1.8

Diffusion

$D_{L_{CO}}$	25 ml/min/mm Hg
$D_{L_{O_2}}$	31 ml/min/mm Hg

Ventilation/blood flow

$\dot{V}_A/\dot{Q}_C$	0.8
$\dot{Q}_s/\dot{Q}_t$	Less than 7%
V_D/V_T	0.3
$P_{a_{O_2}}$	95 mm Hg
Percent saturation	97%
$P_{a_{CO_2}}$	40 mm Hg
pH	7.40

PREDICTION REGRESSIONS FOR PULMONARY FUNCTION TESTS (all values BTPS unless otherwise stated)[*]

TEST	FORMULA	SD	SOURCE
Vital capacity (ml)			
Males	$52.4H - 22.0A - 3600$	580	1
	$48.1H - 20.0A - 2810$	500	2
	$60.4H - 33.2A - 4437$	–	3
Females	$54.5H - 10.5A - 5120$	498	4
	$40.4H - 22.0A - 2350$	400	2
	$48.2H - 17.8A - 3861$	–	3

---

[*]H is height in centimeters; A is age in years; W is weight in kilograms; SD is the standard deviation.

*Functional
residual
capacity (ml)*

Males	$57.8H + 16.0A - 40.0W - 4240$	610	5
Females	$55.9H - 30.0W - 4910$	450	5

*Residual
volume (ml)*

Males	$21.6H + 23.9A - 16.3W - 1680$	415	5
Females	$29.3H + 7.6A - 3730$	348	5

*Total lung
capacity (ml)*

Males	$75.6H - 18.5W - 4690$	730	5
Females	$73.1H - 16.3A - 6280$	522	5

FVC (L)

Males	$0.052H - 0.022A - 3.60$	0.58	1
	$0.148H_{in} - 0.025A - 4.241$	0.74	6
Females	$0.115H_{in} - 0.024A - 2.852$	0.52	6
	$0.0508H - 0.032A - 3.02$	0.52	7

$FEV_{0.5}$ (L)

Males	$0.24 + 0.02H - 0.024A$	0.51	1

$FEV_{1.0}$ (L)

Males	$-1.59 - 0.028A + 0.037H$	0.52	1
	$0.092H_{in} - 0.032A - 1.260$	0.55	6
Females	$0.089H_{in} - 0.025A - 1.932$	0.47	6
	$-0.62 - 0.022A + 0.025H$	0.40	8

*$FEF_{200-1200}$
(L/sec)*

Males	$0.109H_{in} - 0.047A + 2.010$	1.66	6
Females	$0.145H_{in} - 0.036A - 2.532$	1.19	6

*$FEF_{25\%-75\%}$
(L/sec)*

Males	$0.047H_{in} - 0.045A + 2.513$	1.12	6
Females	$0.060H_{in} - 0.030A + 0.551$	0.80	6

*Peak flow,
expiratory
(L/min)*

Males	$(3.95 - 0.0151A)H$	—	9
Females	$(2.93 - 0.0072A)H$	—	9

MVV (L/min)

Males	$(86.5 - 0.522A)S^\circ$	—	10
Females	$(71.3 - 0.474A)S^\circ$	—	10

CV/VC %

Males	$0.357A + 0.562$	4.15	11
Females	$0.293A + 2.812$	4.90	11

CC/TLC %

Males	$0.496A + 14.878$	4.09	11
Females	$0.536A + 14.420$	4.43	11

Viso$\dot{V}$/FVC %

All ages	$0.450A + 4.69$	5.27	12
<50 years	$0.030A + 13.43$	4.31	12

$D_{\text{L}_{\text{CO}}}$

Males	$0.0723H - 0.2793A + 18.167$	—	13
Females	$0.06857H - 0.252A + 15.863$	—	13

°S = Body surface area (m²)

1. Kory, R. C., et al.: Am. J. Med. **30**:243, 1961.
2. Berglund, E., et al.: Acta Med. Scand. **173**:185, 1963.
3. Storstein, O., and Voll, A.: Scand. J. Clin. Lab. Invest. **14**:633, 1962.
4. Anderson, T. W., et al.: Respiration **25**:140, 1968.
5. Grimby, G., and Soderholm, B.: Acta Med. Scand. **173**:199, 1963.
6. Morris, J. F., et al.: Am. Rev. Respir. Dis. **103**:1, 1971.
7. Cotes, J. E., et al.: Br. Med. J. **1**:1016, 1966.
8. Ferris, B. G., Jr., et al.: Am. Rev. Respir. Dis. **91**:252, 1965.
9. Leiner, G. C., et al.: Am. Rev. Respir. Dis. **88:644**, 1963.
10. Baldwin, E., et al.: Medicine (Baltimore) **27**:243, 1948.
11. Buist, S. A., and Ross, B. B.: Am. Rev. Respir. Dis. **107**:744, 1973.
12. Gelb, A. F., et al.: Am. Rev. Respir. Dis. **112**:401, 1975.
13. Bates, D. V., et al.: Med. Serv. J. Can. **18**:211, 1962.

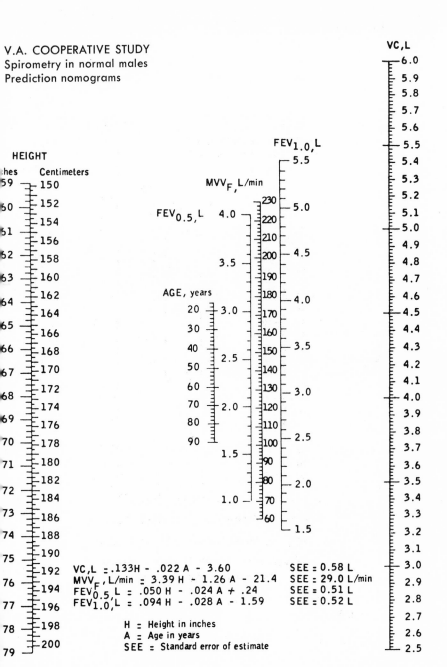

Fig. 1. Clinical spirometry in normal men. (From Kory, R. C., Callahan, R., Boren, H. G., and Syner, J. C.: The Veterans Administration-Army Cooperative Study of Pulmonary Function. I. Clinical spirometry in normal men, AM. J. Med. **30**:243, 1961.)

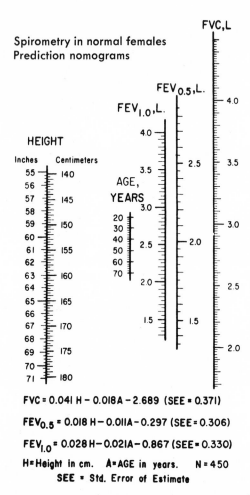

Spirometry in normal females
Prediction nomograms

$FVC = 0.041 H - 0.018A - 2.689$ (SEE = 0.371)

$FEV_{0.5} = 0.018 H - 0.011A - 0.297$ (SEE = 0.306)

$FEV_{1.0} = 0.028 H - 0.021A - 0.867$ (SEE = 0.330)

H = Height in cm.   A = AGE in years.   N = 450
SEE = Std. Error of Estimate

Fig. 2. (Courtesy Dr. Ross C. Kory, Veterans Administration Hospital Tampa, Fla.)

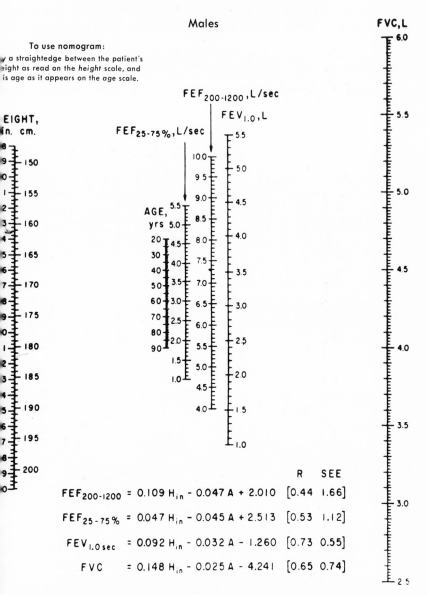

Spirometric standards for normal males (BTPS)

Males

To use nomogram:
y a straightedge between the patient's
eight as read on the *height* scale, and
is age as it appears on the *age* scale.

$$FEF_{200\text{-}1200} = 0.109\,H_{in} - 0.047\,A + 2.010 \quad [0.44 \quad 1.66]$$

$$FEF_{25\text{-}75\%} = 0.047\,H_{in} - 0.045\,A + 2.513 \quad [0.53 \quad 1.12]$$

$$FEV_{1.0\,sec} = 0.092\,H_{in} - 0.032\,A - 1.260 \quad [0.73 \quad 0.55]$$

$$FVC = 0.148\,H_{in} - 0.025\,A - 4.241 \quad [0.65 \quad 0.74]$$

Fig. 3. Prediction nomogram (BTPS), spirometric values in normal males. (From Morris, J. F., Koski, W. A., and Johnson, L. D.: Am. Rev. Resp. Dis. **103**(1):57, 1971.)

Spirometric standards for normal females (BTPS)

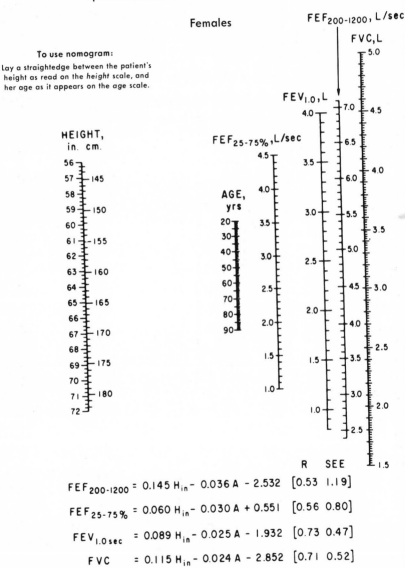

Females

FEF$_{200-1200}$, L/sec

FVC, L

To use nomogram:
Lay a straightedge between the patient's height as read on the *height* scale, and her age as it appears on the *age* scale.

FEV$_{1.0}$, L

HEIGHT,
in. cm.

FEF$_{25-75\%}$, L/sec

AGE,
yrs

R   SEE

$$FEF_{200-1200} = 0.145\,H_{in} - 0.036\,A - 2.532 \quad [0.53 \quad 1.19]$$

$$FEF_{25-75\%} = 0.060\,H_{in} - 0.030\,A + 0.551 \quad [0.56 \quad 0.80]$$

$$FEV_{1.0\,sec} = 0.089\,H_{in} - 0.025\,A - 1.932 \quad [0.73 \quad 0.47]$$

$$FVC = 0.115\,H_{in} - 0.024\,A - 2.852 \quad [0.71 \quad 0.52]$$

Fig. 4. Prediction nomogram (BTPS), spirometric values in normal females. (From Morris, J. F., Koski, W. A., and Johnson, L. C.: Am. Rev. Resp. Dis. **103**(1):57, 1971.)

NORMAL VALUES FOR PULMONARY FUNCTION STUDIES IN CHILDREN*
(all values BTPS; ranges 95% confidence limits)

Age (yr)	Newborn	6	10	14	18	
					♂	♀
Length or height (cm)	51	115	138	160	175	163
Vital capacity (L)	0.14	1.0-1.8	1.7-2.9	2.6-4.5	3.4-6.3	2.7-4.8
Total lung capacity (L)	0.18	1.4-2.3	2.2-3.8	3.5-6.0	4.4-7.6	3.6-6.2
RV/TLC × 100	–	14-34	14-34	14-34	14-34	14-34
MVV (L/min)	–	30-60	42-106	65-140	90-175	62-147
Peak flow, expiratory (L/min)	7.1-10	130-236	217-391	294-534	370-770	295-535
Compliance (ml/cm H_2O)	1-10	32-96	46-142	64-194	78-245	67-204
Airway resistance (cm H_2O/L/sec)	4-41	3-14	2-9	2-6	1-5	2-6
Anatomic dead space (ml)	5.6-12.8	40-78	59-120	84-170	105-205	82-162

*Modified from Cook, C. D. In Nelson, W. E., Vaughan, V. C., III, and McKay, R. J., editors: Textbook of pediatrics, ed. 9, Philadelphia, 1969, W. B. Saunders Co., p. 873.

SUMMARY CURVES FOR PREDICTING
NORMAL VALUES IN CHILDREN

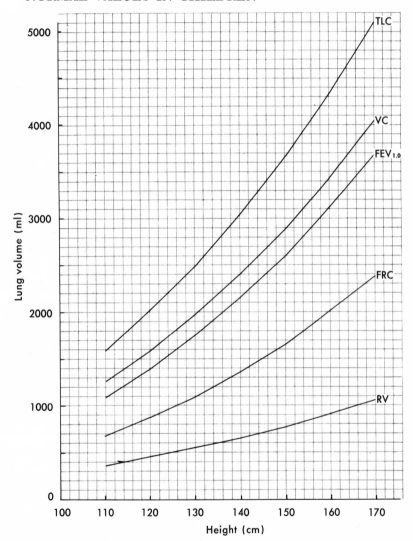

Fig. 5. Summary curves for lung volumes, in ml, for *boys*, as a function of height in cm. Summary curves are derived from regression equations from several different studies. (From Polgar, G., and Promadhat, V.: Pulmonary function testing in children, Philadelphia, 1971, W. B. Saunders Co., p. 209.)

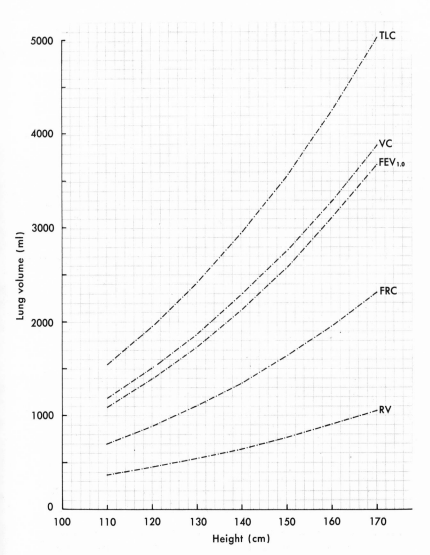

Fig. 6. Summary curves for lung volumes, in ml, for *girls*, as a function of height in cm. Summary curves are derived from regression equations from several different studies. (From Polgar, G., and Promadhat, V.: Pulmonary function testing in children, Philadelphia, 1971, W. B. Saunders Co., p. 210.)

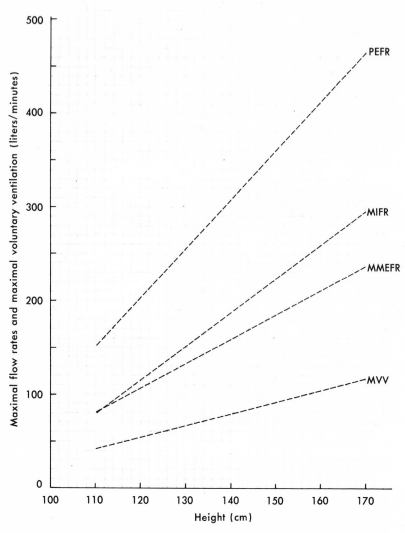

Fig. 7. Summary curves for maximal midexpiratory flow rate ($FEF_{25\%-75\%}$), peak expiratory flow rate (PEFR), maximal voluntary ventilation (MVV), and maximal inspiratory flow rate (MIFR) in L/min, as a function of height for *boys and girls*. Summary curves are derived from regression equations from several different studies. (From Polgar, G., and Promadhat, V.: Pulmonary function testing in children, Philadelphia, 1971, W. B. Saunders Co., p. 211.)

FACTORS FOR CONVERTING GAS VOLUMES FROM ROOM TEMPERATURE TO BTPS

$$\text{Volume (BTPS)} = \text{Volume (ATPS)} \times \frac{P_B - P_{H_2O}}{P_B - 47} \times \frac{310}{273 + T}$$

where

P_B = Barometric pressure, mm Hg
P_{H_2O} = Vapor pressure of water at spirometer temperature
T   = Temperature centigrade
47   = Vapor pressure of water at 37° C
310 = Absolute body temperature

Most of the factors of this equation can be combined to give an approximate value for a conversion factor; local barometric pressure causes slight differences.

Conversion factor	Gas temperature (centigrade)
1.114	18
1.111	19
1.102	20
1.096	21
1.091	22
1.085	23
1.080	24
1.075	25
1.068	26
1.063	27
1.057	28
1.051	29
1.045	30
1.039	31
1.032	32
1.026	33
1.020	34
1.014	35
1.007	36
1.000	37

SYMBOLS AND ABBREVIATIONS USED IN PULMONARY FUNCTION TESTING

LUNG VOLUME	COMPARTMENTS
VC	Vital capacity
IC	Inspiratory capacity
IRV	Inspiratory reserve volume
ERV	Expiratory reserve volume (FRC − RV)
FRC	Functional residual capacity (ERV + RV)
RV	Residual volume
TLC	Total lung capacity (VC + RV)
RV/TLC %	Residual volume to total lung capacity ratio expressed as a percentage
CV	Closing volume
CV/VC %	Closing volume to vital capacity ratio expressed as a percentage
CC	Closing capacity
CC/TLC %	Closing capacity to total lung capacity ratio expressed as a percentage
V_T	Tidal volume
V_A	Alveolar volume
V_D	Dead space volume
V_L	Actual lung volume

VENTILATION

$\dot{V}_E$	Expired volume per minute (BTPS)
$\dot{V}_A$	Alveolar ventilation per minute (BTPS)
$\dot{V}_D$	Dead space ventilation per minute (BTPS)
$\dot{V}_{O_2}$	Oxygen consumption per minute (STPD)
METS	Multiples of the resting oxygen uptake
$\dot{V}_{CO_2}$	Carbon dioxide production per minute (STPD)
f	Respiratory rate per minute
V_D/V_T	Ratio of dead space to tidal volume

SPIROMETRY

FVC	Forced vital capacity with maximally forced expiratory effort
FIVC	Forced inspiratory vital capacity with maximally forced inspiratory effort
FEV_T	Forced expiratory volume for a specific interval T.
FEV_T/FVC %	Forced expiratory volume to forced vital capacity ratio expressed as a percentage

FEF_x — Forced expiratory flow related to some specific portion of the FVC, denoted as subscript x, referring to the amount of FVC already exhaled at the time of measurement

$FEF_{200-1200}$ — Forced expiratory flow between 200 ml and 1200 ml of the FVC (formerly the MEFR)

$FEF_{25\%-75\%}$ — Forced expiratory flow during the middle half of the FVC (formerly the MMF)

PEFR — Peak expiratory flow rate

MEFV — Maximum expiratory flow-volume curve

$\dot{V}_{max_X}$ — Forced expiratory flow related to the actual volume of the lung denoted by subscript X, which refers to the amount of lung volume remaining when measurement is made

Viso$\dot{V}$ — Volume of isoflow

MVV_x — Maximal voluntary ventilation as the volume of air expired in a specified interval, denoted by subscript x (formerly the MBC)

MECHANICS

C — Compliance, volume change per unit of pressure change

C_{dyn} — Dynamic compliance, measured during breathing

C_{st} — Static compliance, measured during periods of no airflow

C/V_L — Specific compliance

FDC — Frequency dependence of compliance $C_{dyn}/C_{st} \times 100$)

R_{aw} — Airway resistance, pressure per unit flow

G_{aw} — Airway conductance, flow per unit of pressure $(1/R_{aw})$

R_{aw}/V_L — Specific resistance

G_{aw}/V_L — Specific conductance

KPM — Kilopound-meters, a unit of power output

DISTRIBUTION

$\Delta N_{2_{750-1250}}$ — Change in percent N_2 over the 750 to 1250 ml portion of the SBN_2 test

SBN_2 — Single-breath nitrogen elimination

Slope of Phase III — Slope of best-fit line through alveolar portion of the SBN_2 from 30% of VC to onset of Phase IV

IDI — Index of distribution of inspired gas (from 7-minute N_2 test)

DIFFUSION

$D_{L_{CO}}$	Diffusing capacity for carbon monoxide
$1/D_m$	Diffusion resistance of the alveolocapillary membrane
$1/\theta V_c$	Diffusion resistance of the red cell and Hb reaction rate
D_L/V_A	Specific diffusion per unit of alveolar lung volume

BLOOD GASES

$P_{A_{O_2}}$	Alveolar oxygen tension
$P_{a_{O_2}}$	Arterial oxygen tension
$S_{a_{O_2}}$	Arterial oxygen saturation
$C_{a_{O_2}}$	Arterial oxygen content
$P_{\bar{v}_{O_2}}$	Mixed venous oxygen tension
$C_{\bar{v}_{O_2}}$	Mixed venous oxygen content
$P_{A_{CO_2}}$	Alveolar carbon dioxide tension
$P_{a_{CO_2}}$	Arterial carbon dioxide tension
$C(a-v)O_2$	Arterial-venous O_2 content difference
$P(A-a)O_2$	Alveolar-arterial O_2 tension difference
pH	Negative logarithm of the H^+ concentration used as a positive number
HCO_3^-	Plasma bicarbonate concentration

GENERAL SYMBOLS

P	Pressure, blood or gas
V	Gas volume
$\dot{V}$	Gas volume per unit time, or flow
F	Fractional concentration of gas
I	Inspired
E	Expired
A	Alveolar
T	Tidal
D	Dead space
$\dot{Q}$	Blood volume
Q	Blood flow
C	Content in blood
S	Saturation
a	Arterial
c	Capillary
v	Venous
$\bar{v}$	Mixed venous
BTPS	Body temperature, saturated with water vapor, body pressure
ATPS	Ambient temperature, pressure, saturated with water vapor
STPD	0°C, 760 mm Hg, dry

MINIMAL SPIROMETRY STANDARDS*

Test	Range/accuracy (BTPS) (liter)	Flow range (L/sec)	Time (sec)	Resistance/back pressure	Test signals
VC	7 L/± 3% of reading or 50 ml, whichever is greater	0-12	60		Calibrated syringe
FVC	7 L/± 3% of reading or 50 ml, whichever is greater	0-12	10.0		2 simulated FVC signals in range (1) FVC = 5 L, t = 0.4 sec; (2) FVC = 3.5 L, t = 2.4 sec
FEV_T†	7 L/± 3% of reading or 50 ml, whichever is greater	0-12	t	Less than 1.5 cm H_2O/L/ sec at 12.0 L/sec flow	Same as FVC
$FEF_{25-75\%}$	7 L/± 5% of reading or 0.1 L/sec, whichever is greater	0-12	10.0	Same as FEV_T	Same as FVC
Flow ($\dot{V}$)	12 L/sec/± 5% of reading or 0.2 L/sec, whichever is greater	0-12	10.0	Same as FEV_T	Manufacturer proof
MVV	Sine wave 250 L/min at 2 L to ± 5% of reading	0-12 ±5%	12-15 ±3%	Less than ± 10 cm H_2O at 2 L V_T, 2.0 Hz	Sine wave pump 0-8 Hz ± 10% at 12 L/sec

*Summarized from *Workshop on Standardization of Spirometry*, sponsored by the American Thoracic Society, Snowbird, Utah, 1977.

†Determination of the "start of test" interval must be made by backward extrapolation of the initial part of the volume-time curve to a point of intersection with the volume baseline.

SOME USEFUL EQUATIONS
Alveolar air equation

It is often necessary to ascertain the composition of alveolar gas. Estimations of the partial pressure of CO_2, N_2, and H_2O can be done rather easily, but the P_{AO_2} is somewhat more difficult to obtain. The most practical application of the alveolar air equation is the determination of alveolar oxygen tension as required for calculation of the percent shunt. The formula for the alveolar air equation is as follows:

$$P_{AO_2} = P_{IO_2} - P_{ACO_2}\left(F_{IO_2} + \frac{1 - F_{IO_2}}{R}\right)$$

where

P_{IO_2} = Partial pressure of O_2 in inspired gas
P_{ACO_2} = Alveolar P_{CO_2} (assumed equal to arterial P_{CO_2})
F_{IO_2} = Fraction of O_2 in inspired gas
R = Respiratory exchange ratio ($\dot{V}_{CO_2}/\dot{V}_{O_2}$)

If the respiratory exchange ratio (R) were 1.0, the entire factor in parentheses would become one and could be deleted. But since the body absorbs more O_2 than it produces CO_2, R is usually less than 1.0 The P_{IO_2} must be calculated from the barometric pressure and corrected to saturation at body temperature by subtracting 47 mm Hg. R usually varies between 0.70 and 1.00 and can usually be assumed to be about 0.80.

Poiseuille's law

Poiseuille's law describes the flow of gas through a tube. The law has many applications in pulmonary physiology, notably insofar as it applies to gas flow through the conducting airways and as it is utilized in pneumotachography. The law is stated thus:

$$\Delta P = \frac{\dot{V}8\eta l}{\pi r^4}$$

where

ΔP = Change in pressure from one end of the tube to the other
$\dot{V}$ = Flow through the tube
η = Coefficient of viscosity of the gas

l = Length of the tube
r = Radius of the tube

The equation can be rearranged thus:

$$\frac{\Delta P}{\dot V} = \frac{8\eta l}{\pi r^4}$$

Here the relationship between the pressure difference at the ends of the tube and the flow through the tube, which defines *resistance*, is equated to the remaining variables, notably the length and radius of the tube. It should be noted that the resistance varies directly with the length of the conducting tube and inversely with the radius. A twofold increase in the length of the tube doubles the resistance, whereas a reduction of the radius by half increases the pressure differential sixteen times. In the airways, abnormal narrowing by mucous secretions or functional lesions can cause significant increases in airway resistance. Since Poiseuille's law holds true for any round tube in which laminar flow is possible, the principle of pneumotachography is based directly on this law. Because the length and radius of a pneumotach flow tube remain constant and the viscosity of respiratory gases varies only slightly, all the variables in Poiseuille's equation can be reduced to a constant except ΔP and $\dot V$. By rearranging:

$$\dot V = \frac{\Delta P}{K_R}$$

where

K_R = Resistance constant

From this equation it is obvious that all that is necessary to measure the flow ($\dot V$) is a means of determining the pressure differential; this is easily accomplished by means of pressure transducers.

Thoracic gas volume equation

Measurement of the thoracic gas volume with the body plethysmograph is based on Boyle's law:

$$P_1 V_1 = P_2 V_2$$

or

$$P_1V_1 = (P_1 + \Delta P)(V_1 + \Delta V)$$

Simplifying

$$P_1\Delta V + V_1\Delta P + \Delta V\Delta P = 0$$

where

P_1 = Initial pressure in the lungs (713 mm Hg or 970 cm H_2O)
V_1 = V_{TG} or thoracic gas volume
ΔV = Change in lung volume
ΔP = Change in lung pressure

Solving for V_1:

$$V_1 = -\frac{\Delta V}{\Delta P}(P_1 + \Delta P)$$

Since ΔP is small compared with P_1, $P_1 + \Delta P \cong P_1$ and therefore:

$$V_1 = -\frac{P_1(\Delta V)}{\Delta P}$$

In terms of the plethysmographic method (and disregarding the sign):

$$V_{TG} = 970\frac{(\Delta V)}{(\Delta P)}$$

The slope recorded on the oscilloscope is the change in mouth pressure per unit change in box volume, $\frac{(\Delta P)}{(\Delta V)}$ or V_{TG}, as the subject breathes against an occluded airway. The equation then becomes:

$$V_{TG} = \frac{970}{\lambda V_{TG}}$$

This is the working form of the equation after box and pressure calibrations have been included. Simple measurement of the slope of the trace allows rapid calculation of V_{TG}.

Fick's law of diffusion (modified)

In reference to gas exchange across a membrane, Fick's law states that:

$$\dot{V}_{gas} = \frac{A}{T} \times D \times (P_1 - P_2)$$

where

A	= Area of the membrane
T	= Thickness of the membrane
$P_1 - P_2$	= Pressure gradient across the membrane
D	= Diffusion constant

D is related to the molecular weight and solubility of the gas to which it refers by:

$$D \propto \frac{\text{Solubility}}{\sqrt{\text{Mol. wt.}}}$$

Since A and T remain constant in the lung system:

$$D_L \propto \frac{\dot{V}_{gas}}{P_A - P_c}$$

where

D_L	= Diffusion constant for the lung
P_A	= Alveolar gas pressure
P_c	= Capillary gas pressure

When D_L is measured with carbon monoxide, the capillary partial pressure is assumed to be zero, thus:

$$D_L = \frac{\dot{V}_{CO}}{P_{A_{CO}}}$$

All of the carbon monoxide methods of measuring D_L use this basic equation. The single-breath and steady state methods differ in that the former measures $\dot{V}_{CO}$ during breath holding, while the latter measures it during "normal" breathing. The steady state methods vary by the way in which they measure $P_{A_{CO}}$.

Fick principle (cardiac output determination)

The Fick principle relates oxygen consumption ($\dot{V}_{O_2}$) to arterial-venous oxygen content difference ($C[a\text{-}v]O_2$) to determine cardiac output ($\dot{Q}$):

$$\dot{Q} = \frac{\dot{V}_{O_2}}{C_aO_2 - C_{\bar{v}}O_2}$$

This equation forms the basis for determining various fractions of the cardiac output, namely the shunt fraction (Q_s) and the fraction participating in ideal gas exchange (Q_c). The relationship between the shunt fraction (Q_s) and the total cardiac output (Q_t) can be expressed as a ratio using the concept of oxygen content differences:

$$\frac{\dot{Q}_s}{\dot{Q}_t} = \frac{C_{\bar{c}}O_2 - C_aO_2}{C_{\bar{c}}O_2 - C_{\bar{v}}O_2}$$

where

$C_cO_2 - C_aO_2 =$ Content difference between pulmonary end-capillary blood, C_cO_2, and arterial blood, C_aO_2, which increases when blood passes through the the pulmonary system without coming into contact with alveolar gas (a shunt)

$C_{\bar{c}}O_2 - C_{\bar{v}}O_2 =$ Content difference between blood returning to the lungs by way of the pulmonary artery and the pulmonary end-capillary blood; the total change reflecting the arterialization of mixed venous blood

In a system in which all blood equilibrates with alveolar gas, C_cO_2 and C_aO_2 become identical, no matter what the value of the denominator, so that the ratio becomes zero and the shunt must be zero. As more blood fails to equilibrate, the numerator becomes larger in relation to the denominator and is reflected by an increased $\dot{Q}_s/\dot{Q}_t$.

Since true pulmonary end-capillary oxygen content, C_cO_2, is practically impossible to sample and represents a mathematical entity rather than an actual phenomenon, a modified form of the equation is used clinically (as described in Chapter 6):

$$\frac{\dot{Q}_s}{\dot{Q}_t} = \frac{(P_{A_{O_2}} - P_{a_{O_2}})(0.0031)}{(C[a\text{-}v]O_2) + (P_{A_{O_2}} - P_{a_{O_2}})(0.0031)}$$

where

$P_{A_{O_2}} - P_{a_{O_2}}$ = *Tension* difference of oxygen between the alveoli and arterial blood

0.0031 = Solubility factor to convert O_2 tension to volumes percent

The equation is implemented by having the subject breath 100% O_2 long enough to completely saturate the hemoglobin ($P_{a_{O_2}}$ greater than 150 mm Hg). Therefore the only difference between pulmonary end-capillary blood (assumed to be in equilibrium with the $P_{A_{O_2}}$) and arterial blood exists in the difference in oxygen content in the dissolved form. Again this is related to the normal a-v content difference ($C[a\text{-}v]O_2$) plus the actual dissolved content difference, denoted by the same term in both numerator and denominator. A ratio is thus derived between the content difference of shunted blood and the total content difference, in this case determined by using dissolved oxygen differences. $P_{A_{O_2}}$ is determined by the alveolar air equation outlined above.

Oxygen consumption, CO_2 production, and respiratory quotient

Oxygen consumption, $\dot{V}_{O_2}$, is determined by calculating the difference between the amount of O_2 inhaled and exhaled:

$$\dot{V}_{O_2}(STPD) = (\dot{V}_I \times F_{I_{O_2}}) - (\dot{V}_E \times F_{E_{O_2}})$$

where

$\dot{V}_I$ = Volume inspired per minute
$\dot{V}_E$ = Volume expired per minute
$F_{I_{O_2}}$ = Fractional concentration of inspired oxygen
$F_{E_{O_2}}$ = Fractional concentration of expired oxygen

Presuming that inspired and expired volumes are equal, the equation can be simplified:

$$\dot{V}_{O_2} = \dot{V}_E \times (F_{I_{O_2}} - F_{E_{O_2}})$$

CO_2 production is determined similarly:

$$\dot{V}_{CO_2} \text{ (STPD)} = \dot{V}_E \times (F_{ECO_2} - F_{ICO_2})$$

Since the fractional concentration of CO_2 in inspired air is only 0.0004 the equation becomes:

$$\dot{V}_{CO_2} = \dot{V}_E \times (F_{ECO_2} - 0.0004$$

The respiratory quotient, R, represents the ratio of CO_2 production to O_2 consumption and can be determined by combining the above equations:

$$R = \frac{\dot{V}_{CO_2}}{\dot{V}_{O_2}} = \frac{\dot{V}_E \times (F_{ECO_2} - F_{ICO_2})}{\dot{V}_E \times (F_{IO_2} - F_{EO_2})}$$

or simplifying:

$$R = \frac{F_{ECO_2} - F_{ICO_2}}{F_{IO_2} - F_{EO_2}}$$

SAMPLE CALCULATIONS
Open-circuit FRC determination (N_2 washout) (refer to p. 4)

FRC: Unknown
%N_2 final: 6% (0.06 as a fraction)
Vol. expired: 27.5 L
%N_2 alveolar: 75% (0.75 as a fraction)
Test time (T): 7 minutes
Blood/tissue N_2 washout factor: 0.04 L/min (correction factor)
Spirometer/breathing circuit V_D: 1.0 L
Spirometer temp.: 24°C

1. $FRC = \dfrac{\%N_2 \text{ final} \times (\text{vol. expired} + \text{dead space})}{\%N_2 \text{ alveolar}} -$

$(T \times N_2 \text{ correction})$

2. $= \dfrac{0.06 \times (27.5 \text{ L} + 1.0 \text{ L})}{0.75} - (7.0 \text{ min} \times 0.04 \text{ L/min})$

3. $= \dfrac{0.06 \times 28.5 \text{ L}}{0.75} - (0.28\text{L})$

4. $= \dfrac{1.71 \text{ L}}{0.75} - (0.28 \text{ L})$

5. $= 2.28 \text{ L} - 0.28 \text{ L}$

6. FRC = 2.00 L (ATPS)

This value is ATPS and must be corrected to BTPS. The spirometer temperature was 24°C; thus using the appropriate correction factor from p. 145:

7. FRC (BTPS) = 2.00 L × 1.08

8. FRC (BTPS) = 2.16

Closed-circuit FRC determination (helium dilution) (refer to p. 6)

FRC: Unknown
He added: 0.5 L
$\%He_{initial}$: 9.5% (0.095 as a fraction)
$\%He_{final}$: 5.5% (0.055 as a fraction)
He absorption correction: 0.1 L
Spirometer temp.: 24°C

1. $FRC = \left[\dfrac{(\%He_{initial} - \%He_{final})}{\%He_{final}} \times \text{Initial volume} \right] -$

$\qquad\qquad\qquad\qquad\qquad\qquad\qquad$ He absorption correction

2. Initial volume $= \dfrac{\text{He added}}{\%He_{initial}}$
   (spirometer +
   circuitry)

$$= \frac{0.5\ L}{0.095}$$

$$= 5.26\ L$$

3. $FRC = \left[\dfrac{(0.095 - 0.055)}{0.055} \times 5.26\ L \right] - 0.1\ L$

4. $\qquad = (0.73 \times 5.26\ L) - 0.1\ L$

5. $\qquad = 3.84\ L - 0.1\ L$

6. FRC = 3.74 L (ATPS)

Correcting to BTPS with appropriate correction factor from p. 145:

7. FRC (BTPS) = 3.74 L × 1.08

8. FRC (BTPS) = 4.04 L

Single-breath D_{LCO} (refer to Chapter 5)

Vol. inspired: 4.0 L
Breath hold time ($t_2 - t_1$): 10.0 sec

$F_{I_{CO}}$: 0.3% (0.003 as a fraction); also $F_{A_{CO_{t_1}}}$

$F_{A_{CO_{t_2}}}$: 0.125% (0.00125 as a fraction)

$F_{I_{He}}$: 10.0% (0.10 as a fraction)

$F_{E_{He}}$: 7.5% (0.075 as a fraction)

P_B: 760 mm Hg

Spirometer temp.: 25°C

1. $D_{L_{CO}}SB = \dfrac{V_A \times 60}{(P_B - 47)(t_2 - t_1)} \times Ln \dfrac{(F_{A_{CO_{t_1}}})}{(F_{A_{CO_{t_2}}})}$

2. $V_A = \dfrac{\text{Vol. inspired}}{F_{E_{He}}/F_{I_{He}}}$

$= \dfrac{4.0\ L}{0.075/0.10} = 5.33\ L\ (5333\ ml)$

3. $F_{A_{CO_{t_1}}} = F_{I_{CO}} \times F_{E_{He}}/F_{I_{He}}$

$= 0.003 \times 0.075/0.10 = .0025$

4. $D_{L_{CO}}SB = \dfrac{5333\ ml \times 60}{(713) \times (10.0)} \times Ln \dfrac{(0.0025)}{(0.00125)}$

5. $= \dfrac{319.980}{7130} \times Ln\ (2.0)$

6. $= 44.9\ ml/min/mm\ Hg \times (0.6931)$

7. $= 31.10\ ml\ CO/min/mm\ Hg\ (ATPS)$

This value is ATPS and is normally converted to STPD (0°C, 760 mm Hg, dry). The correction factor can be calculated:

8. $\dfrac{273}{273 + T°C} \times \dfrac{P_B - P_{H_2O}\ T°C}{760} = \text{correction factor}$

where

$T°C$ = Spirometer temperature

$P_{H_2O}T°C$ = Partial pressure of water vapor at the spirometer temperature (in this case: 24 mm Hg at 25°C)

9. $\dfrac{273}{273 + 25} \times \dfrac{760 - 24}{760} = \text{correction factor}$

10. $0.916 \times 0.968 = 0.887$

11. $(31.10\ ml\ CO/min/mm\ Hg) \times (0.887) = 27.6\ ml\ CO\ (STPD)/min/mm\ Hg$

Index